Caring for Patients
from Different Cultures

Second Edition

Caring for Patients from Different Cultures

Case Studies
from American Hospitals

SECOND EDITION

Geri-Ann Galanti

PENN

University of Pennsylvania Press

Philadelphia

Published by
University of Pennsylvania Press
Philadelphia, Pennsylvania 19104-6097

Library of Congress Cataloging-in-Publication Data

Galanti, Geri-Ann.
    Caring for patients from different cultures : case studies from
  American hospitals / Geri-Ann Galanti. —2nd ed.
       p.   cm.
    Includes bibliographical references and index.
    ISBN 0-8122-1608-3 (pbk. : alk. paper)
    1. Transcultural nursing—Case studies. 2. Transcultural medical care—Case
  studies. 3. Hospital care—Psycological aspects—Case studies. 4. Ethnopsychology—
  Case studies. I. Title.
  RT86.54.G35   1997
  610.73—dc20   96-35530
                                                                        CIP

. . . in memory of my brother, Bryan Galanti . . .

You are not forgotten

Contents

Preface

Whenever I see a second edition of a book, I ask, "Why?" It is often because new research has revealed new data or new theories have shed light on earlier research. Neither exactly accounts for the writing of this edition, however. Cultures have not changed much since the first edition came out in 1991. So why write another?

Because in the years since the first edition was published, I have done a lot more teaching and lecturing and have a better sense of what information health care providers need. The scope of my research broadened when one of the programs I teach for—the Division of Nursing at California State University, Dominguez Hills—went national via cable television through Mind Extension University, giving me access to nurses all over the country. I also began conducting workshops on cultural diversity at hospitals and conferences. As a result, I gained a greater sense of the concerns of the people on the front lines—the nurses, physicians, managers, aides, and other health care providers. I was delighted to get much positive feedback on my book, but I saw that additional material would be helpful. So I collected more cases and reorganized the book, adding several new chapters. I hope that the changes will make the book even more useful for its readers.

As before, the credit for the book belongs to the thousands of nurses and other health care professionals who over the years have shared with me the frustration of dealing with the huge ethnic populations in the United States. When I first began teaching nursing classes, I was incredibly idealistic. I thought I could give the students the knowledge they would need to provide ethnically appropriate care. I found, however, that most nurses are overworked and have little time to make adjustments for ethnic differences. They work in the "real world," not an academically idealized version of it. Were my classes of no value, then, beyond mere curiosity?

Fortunately, no. I found I could significantly reduce the nurses' stress by explaining why their patients acted as they did. They were not deliberately trying to irritate the staff; they were simply behaving according to their customs. Now, when people ask me what I do, I explain that I teach health care providers why their patients are *interesting* rather than annoying. It makes a difference.

Unlike many books on health care, this one spends little time on theoretical issues. Over the years, I have found that the most effective way to make a point is to tell a story. People remember anecdotes much better than they do dry facts and theories. Theories that grow out of stories are much easier to grasp and retain than ones presented in a vacuum. I was fortunate in having a constant source of anecdotes—my students. They were working in the field, observing the actual problems that occur as a result of cultural differences. The cases that one class shared with me, I in turn shared with the next.

The general organization of the book is identical to that of the first edition. The first chapter covers basic theoretical concepts. The rest of the book contains the best of the hundreds of incidents of conflict and misunderstanding that my students experienced. I have tried to give solutions or ways to avoid problems whenever possible, although it is not always feasible. In every case, however, I have attempted to explain why people acted the way they did. I hope that the book will help readers to see things through the eyes of people from cultures that are different from theirs. For me, that is the greatest contribution anthropology can make to the world.

My only fear is that people of different ethnic groups will read this book and feel they have been presented in a bad light or that the individual in the case described is a poor representative of his or her ethnic group. Such accusations would not be entirely unjustified. I have chosen cases that created the greatest trouble for the hospital staff, and the individuals involved may not represent the best of their ethnic groups. I have tried to choose examples of behavior that reflect cultural values or customs, even if the behavior is an extreme version. It is my intention to promote understanding, not prejudice. (Troublesome members of my own ethnic group are also well represented here.) I will make a blanket apology at the outset, lest I offend anyone. Truly, no offense is meant.

I should also add that I intended no disrespect to any members of the health care profession. Some of the nurses depicted, and many of the physicians, do not come across as very admirable. Individuals should not be taken to represent all members of that group. Perhaps doctors appear more frequently in a negative light due to the inherent conflict between nursing and medicine—and the fact that nurses provided me with most of the cases.

The book is organized into thirteen chapters. The first introduces the

basic relevant anthropological concepts, and the following eleven are arranged according to topic: communication; pain; religion and beliefs;
diet; family; men and women; staff relations; birth; death; mental health;
and folk medicine. The final chapter is a brief summary. I chose a topi-
cal organization rather than one by ethnic group, both to be in keeping
with standard nursing texts and because I felt it was more suitable for
making theoretical points. The chapter divisions, however, are somewhat
arbitrary. There may be material in one chapter that could just as easily
fit into another. In such cases, I have referred the reader to related material in other chapters. Some material did not fit well into any chapter
but did not warrant a separate one. Life does not always fit into neat
categories.

As in the first edition, the numbers in the first index refer to *case study
numbers* (found in the margins) rather than page numbers. I have
changed the organization of this index to a more standardized format.
In the original edition, it was done by topic. It seemed like a good idea
at the time, but frankly, I didn't find it very useful. In this edition, the
material is indexed by ethnic group and then just alphabetically. I have
also added a second index by page number

Unlike most books, this one can be read in almost any order, a few
pages at a time, although the first chapter should be read first. Each case
is self-contained and can be understood on its own.

I decided to use names for all the patients and hospital staff in the
various case studies; it makes the stories more accessible. I tried to use
ethnically appropriate names whenever possible. All names are fictitious.
If I inadvertently used someone's real name, it was accidental. I used first
names for the nurses and last names for the doctors to reflect their usage
in practice. For the patients, I generally used first names for individuals
under thirty and last names for those older, simply to provide variety.

I should also note that the terms "African American" and "Black" are
used interchangeably throughout the book. Both are in common usage
at the time of writing, and each reflects the preferences of different
individuals.

The major goal of the book is to help health care professionals recognize the cultural dimensions of problems that occur in hospitals between
and among patients, their families, and staff. Obviously, not every possible problem can be documented. There is no easy "recipe" for solving
problems; each individual and situation is different. My hope is that this
book will give the reader some idea of the range of cultural behaviors
and the need to understand people's actions from their own cultural
perspective.

The bibliography is intended as a resource guide for those who want to do more research, either out of general interest or to deal with specific problems. It is divided into three subjects: general texts and articles on transcultural nursing and medical anthropology, ethnic groups, and special topics. The list is by no means exhaustive, but it should provide a useful starting point.

Acknowledgments

First, second, and third, I want to thank the hundreds of nurses who generously shared with me the cross-cultural misunderstandings they encountered in their work. Without them, there would be no book. Next, I am indebted to the Division of Nursing at California State University, Dominguez Hills, and the Department of Anthropology at California State University, Los Angeles, where I have taught the courses which gave me access to the nurses who shared their experiences. Next, I want to thank all those who hired me to conduct workshops on cultural diversity. Lecturing is a two-way street; I always learn from those I teach.

I also want to thank my editor at UPP, Patricia Reynolds Smith. Not only do I value her astute suggestions and advice, but I have come to appreciate what a delight she is to work with. I am the only academic I know who actually likes her editor. Thank you, Patricia.

The teachers and mentors whom I acknowledged in the first edition still deserve credit—Robert Edgerton, Allen Johnson, Susan Scrimshaw, and Lowell Sever. Although she doesn't know me, Madeleine Leininger deserves my recognition for creating the field of transcultural nursing.

Without my husband, Donald Sutherland, I could not have written this volume. He originally conceived of the book, as well as made my life easy while I was writing this edition. I am eternally grateful. Thank you, Don, for everything.

I also want to thank my huge Sephardic family. I never realized how different my upbringing was from that of most Americans until I was in college and read the classic article, "The Folk Society," by Robert Redfield. My first reaction was: "The folk society? This sounds just like my family." Being raised in my family gave me greater insight into more traditional cultures as well as surrounding me with the love and security that gave me the courage to make my way in the world.

Finally, I want to thank my friends who, to me, are like family. You make the world a much better place. But please don't keep moving out of town.

Chapter 1
Basic Concepts

If the United States is a melting pot, the cultural stew still has a lot of lumps.

Introduction

What happens when an Iranian doctor and a Filipino nurse treat a Mexican patient? When a Navaho patient calls a medicine man to the hospital? Or when an Anglo nurse refuses to take orders from a Japanese doctor? Generally, the result is confusion and conflict, unless they all have some understanding of cultural differences.

The health care system in the United States has been in a state of crisis for some time. An obvious problem is the cost and apportionment of medical care. A more subtle problem that is beginning to receive attention involves the cultural gap between the medical system and the huge number of ethnic minorities it serves.

The goal of the medical system is to provide optimal care for all patients. In a multiethnic society, this can be accomplished only if the health care providers understand such things as why Asian patients rarely ask for pain medication whereas patients from Mediterranean countries seem to need it for the slightest discomfort, why Middle Easterners will not allow a male physician to examine their women, and that coin rubbing is an Asian form of medical treatment, not a method of child abuse.

This book addresses the cultural differences that create conflicts and misunderstandings and that may result in inferior medical care. First, however, some basic understanding of anthropological principles is required. The remainder of this chapter is devoted to several of the more important concepts. Many will be reviewed in the chapters that follow as well, when the incidents that illustrate the principles are described.

Culture

A basic working definition of culture is that it encompasses beliefs and
behaviors that are learned and shared by members of a group.

A man I know removes his shoes when he enters the house. He has
indoor shoes and outdoor shoes and will not wear one for the other. Is
this a cultural trait or a personal idiosyncrasy? From the information
given, it is impossible to tell. One must know his ethnic background. If
he were Japanese, it would be a cultural trait. He is not. He is a white
Anglo-Saxon Protestant from New York. Thus this trait is a personal idiosyncrasy. For behavior to be cultural, it must be learned and shared by
members of a group. New York WASPs do not make a practice of removing their shoes when entering a house. The Japanese do.

Stereotype Versus Generalization

I will be making many generalizations in this book. They should not be
mistaken for stereotypes. A stereotype and a generalization may appear
similar, but they function very differently. An example is the assumption
that Mexicans have large families. If I meet Rosa, a Mexican woman, and
I say to myself, "Rosa is Mexican; she must have a large family," I am
stereotyping her. But if I think Mexicans often have large families and
wonder whether Rosa does, I am making a generalization.

A stereotype is an ending point. No attempt is made to learn whether
the individual in question fits the statement. Stereotyping patients can
have negative results.

Lily was a forty-eight-year-old woman from the Middle East. She was
in the county hospital to have surgery for gallstones. Sandy, a Mexican
American nurse, was caring for her prior to surgery. Sandy cared for Lily
for three nights and describes them as a nightmare. Lily did nothing
but moan and groan and demand pain medication. She was on the call
light continually. Sandy did her job but resented Lily's behavior. She
chalked it up to Lily's ethnic background—Middle Easterners are often
demanding and express their pain freely and loudly. She looked forward
to Lily's surgery; at last, her gallstones would be removed and she could
go home.

When Sandy returned to work a week later, she learned that Lily had
not had gallstones after all. When the surgeons opened her up, they discovered that cancer had invaded her entire gastrointestinal system. She
died on the operating table. Sandy's heart sank. She had stereotyped Lily
as just another loud, complaining Middle Easterner. It turned out that
she had been moaning and groaning and requesting pain medication,
not because she was Middle Eastern, but because she was riddled with

1

cancer and in excruciating pain. It was an important lesson for Sandy about the dangers of stereotyping.

A generalization, on the other hand, is a beginning point. It indicates common trends, but further information is needed to ascertain whether the statement is appropriate to a particular individual. Generalizations may be inaccurate when applied to specific individuals, but anthropologists do apply generalizations broadly, looking for common patterns, for beliefs and behaviors that are shared by the group. It is important to remember, however, that there are always differences between individuals.

Factors other than innate personality can cause individuals to deviate from the norm for their culture. These factors include the length of time they have spent in the United States, the age at which they came here, their desire to assimilate, whether they live in an ethnic community or an "American" one, whether they came from a rural or urban area, and their level of education. Social and economic class can be even more important than ethnic background. Middle-class Blacks, for example, often have more in common with middle-class Caucasians than with lower-class Blacks.

I have purposely chosen examples of individuals who have not assimilated to a great degree and whose beliefs and behaviors deviate from those expressed in the American health care system. It should not be inferred that all or even most members of these groups will act in the manner described. The ones who are most Westernized do not generally present problems. It is those who adhere to traditional ways that are most likely to, hence their inclusion in this book. It should be remembered, however, that assimilation occurs in unpredictable stages. Individuals may be quite Westernized in some areas but traditional in others.

I will be making many generalizations throughout this book. I will also be lumping together groups that are actually quite distinct from each other. The term "Hispanic" or "Latino" includes people from such diverse cultures as Mexican, Puerto Rican, Argentinian, and Peruvian. "Asian" refers to people from a variety of countries, including China, Japan, Korea, Vietnam, Cambodia, and the Philippines. It is dangerous and inaccurate to think they are all alike. When I do make such generalizations, it is because there are some traits that are fairly consistent across cultures within the designated group. But never forget individual differences.

Also remember, when you come into contact with people from different cultures, that it is often highly offensive to them to be labeled by the wrong country. Many are historical enemies. There is also a tremendous amount of prejudice and stereotyping within each larger culture area. A Chinese student shared that many Chinese think that Vietnamese have prominent cheekbones, Koreans have small eyes, and Japanese are short. These are all seen as characteristics that are inferior to those of the more "beautiful" Chinese. A Chinese person would likely be insulted if mistaken for a Korean, and vice versa. Ethnocentrism is universal, and stereotyping occurs even within ethnic groups.

2   Carla, a half-Mexican nurse, observed that in Mexico those with more European blood often feel superior to those with more Indian heritage. In addition, city people look down somewhat on rural people. It is an insult to call someone "provincial." Those from D.F. (Districto Federal, Mexico City) feel superior to everyone. She, however, prided herself on being immune to all the hierarchical structuring; she firmly believed in the equality of all people.

One day Carla had a patient who was from Mexico. Carla assumed from Mrs. Arroyo's dark skin, black hair, and facial features that she was a Mexican Indian, probably with little education. Carla realized she would have to speak to her rather simply, to make sure that she understood. This was probably her first time in a hospital. She then asked the patient which part of Mexico she was from. Mrs. Arroyo looked Carla directly in the eyes and said, "I'm from D.F. And you?"

Carla, who had never realized her own inherent prejudices, was speechless for a moment. She replied, "My father is from Guanajuato." To which Mrs. Arroyo responded, "Yes, I thought as much. I can always spot you provincial people; you are very different."

There are some lessons to be learned from this incident. One is that most of us, even though we may consider ourselves free of prejudice, probably are not. Another is that even within the same culture, people judge and stereotype each other. Finally, it is always a mistake to stereotype people on the basis of appearance.

Generalizations made in this book about large cultural groups such as Asians or Hispanics may be seen as a way of distinguishing broad geographical groupings from each other while recognizing that there are differences within them. Also, on occasion, the only ethnic identity given for a patient is Asian or Hispanic because more detailed information was not known but the case illustrated a general point common to most cultures within that group.

Prejudice and Discrimination

An important related issue in today's world, given strained inter-ethnic relations, is that of prejudice and discrimination. The long history of slavery in this country, followed by Reconstruction and its aftermath, along with less institutionalized racism, has lead many African Americans to distrust the health care system.

Mr. Harris, a sixty-eight-year-old Black male, was scheduled to have his 3
cancerous prostate removed at a government hospital. Two days after
scheduling the procedure, he called Karen, his nurse, in panic. He had
spoken to several friends about his upcoming surgery, and now wanted
to know about various forms of alternative treatments. Karen spent about
an hour on the phone with him and gave him a great deal of information
as well as phone numbers he could call to learn about other options. She
realized that he was probably overwhelmed and frightened about his
diagnosis.

Right before hanging up, Mr. Harris said, "You know I trust *you*, Karen;
I just don't know if I trust the hospital to take care of me. I have older
friends who were subjected to government studies without knowing it
back in the '40s and '50s." Karen suddenly realized it wasn't just the cancer he feared, but what a white institution might do to him, a Black man.
The experiments done with syphilitic Black men who were left untreated
in order to study the course of the disease are infamous.

It is no wonder that many African Americans are distrustful of hospitals—and white institutions in general. Prejudice and discrimination are
real. Not surprisingly, if you have been a frequent victim of discrimination, you are likely to come to expect it, even, as in the next two cases,
when it is not there.

The patient was a ten-month-old Black male. His hands and feet were 4
tied to the bed to prevent him from pulling out the intravenous lines.
When Mrs. Wilson, his grandmother, saw him tied down, she became
very angry. "How come you got the baby tied down? He's not doing anything. He ain't no trouble. Why don't you untie him? He looks like he
can't move. He ain't no dog!" She had experienced much discrimination
at the hands of whites and perceived her grandson's treatment as a racist
act. Once the nurse explained the purpose of tying the baby down, she
relaxed.

Similarly, during a prenatal exam, an obstetrics resident asked the 5
patient whether she had considered having her tubes tied at the time
of delivery. The patient, Lotty Parker, was a forty-three-year-old Black
woman, pregnant with her twelfth child. Mrs. Parker immediately became angry, saying, "I ain't gonna have no white doctor messin' with my
insides!" The resident may have felt that it was his responsibility to explain increased pregnancy risks after forty, but the Black woman apparently viewed his suggestion as a form of racial genocide. Health care
personnel must be especially sensitive to this issue when dealing with
patients from minority ethnic groups.

There is good reason for African Americans to be wary of the predominantly white health care institution. Prejudice and discrimination
do exist. Unless one has had the experience of being stopped by the po-

lice simply for driving a nice car in a good neighborhood, or been asked by a white salesperson, "Are you sure you can afford it?" when buying a high ticket item, it is difficult to understand what it is like to be the recipient of racial prejudice. We are all individuals and want to be treated as such, but, unfortunately, minorities are often judged simply on the color of their skin.

At the same time, however, years of discrimination may have led some individuals to be acutely sensitive and to perceive prejudice when it does not exist. Health care providers should be aware of this and do what they can to ensure that their words and actions do not unintentionally hurt their patients.

Values

Values are the things we hold as important. Just as each individual holds certain values, each culture promotes different ones. American culture (and I use this term loosely because there are literally hundreds of subcultures within the United States) currently values such things as money, freedom, independence, privacy, health and fitness, and physical appearance.

One way to assess a culture's values is to observe how it punishes people. In the United States wrongdoers are punished by being fined (taking away their *money*) or incarcerated (taking away their *freedom*). The Mbuti pygmies of Africa value social support, and they punish people by ignoring them. The kind of health care provided by the American medical system is often influenced by financial considerations, whereas concern for family, low on the list of "American" values, influences much patient behavior. Hence conflict may develop between health care providers and patients.

In the United States, *independence* is manifested by the desire to move away from home as soon as one is financially able. In many cultures that value family more than independence, adult children rarely move out before marriage and often not thereafter. The health care culture also supports the values of independence and *autonomy* in its efforts to teach self-care and in often giving information only to the patient, excluding other family members.

Privacy is also very important to most Americans, who build fences to separate their houses from each other. The U.S. health care culture tries to provide privacy for patients by limiting visiting hours and offering no sleeping accommodations for visitors. Many non-Anglo patients, however, prefer just the opposite.

Health and *fitness* are popular movements, particularly on the West Coast. There are hundreds of food products labeled "low fat" and "low cholesterol." People can be seen jogging on most city streets, and attendance at gyms is high. This obsession with health leads the medical profession to expect patients to comply with suggestions regarding changes in diet and exercise, assuming that health and fitness is a value shared by all. It is not. Furthermore, what is considered "healthy" varies cross-culturally.

Concern for *physical appearance* is manifested at every magazine stand. There are few women's magazines that do not have articles on the latest diet, makeup, hairdo, and clothing. The incidence of cosmetic surgery for both men and women is at a record high. Surgical techniques are developed to minimize scarring and maintain beauty. What is considered "beautiful," however, is not the same for every culture.

Understanding people's values is the key to understanding their behavior, for our behavior generally reflects our values. A dramatic example occurred in the early 1980s, when a Japanese ship captain was bringing a boatload of cars to the United States. There was a disaster at sea, and the cargo was ruined. The captain had done nothing to cause the disaster, and he could not have prevented it. If an American ship captain had had a similar experience, the first thing he probably would have done when he reached land was call his insurance agent to see who would pay for the damages. The Japanese captain killed himself.

There is obviously a big difference between calling one's insurance agent and killing oneself. The different reactions are dictated by different values. The hypothetical American captain would probably value *money*; his concern would be for the financial loss. The Japanese captain was concerned with his *honor*. As the captain of the ship, he considered himself responsible for the accident. The loss of the cargo meant the loss of his honor. Without honor, he felt he could not live. Committing ritual suicide was the only way for him to regain his honor.

Values influence our everyday behavior as well. Why are you reading this book? Is it because you value knowledge and hope to learn something? Is it because you are required to read it for a course and you value good grades? If so, are you motivated because good grades will get you a better job, and with a better job you will earn more money, and you value money? Nearly everything we do reflects our values on some level.

Values and the American Health Care Culture

One reason for so many conflicts and misunderstandings in hospitals is the great disjunction between the values of the health care culture and that of the patient population.

As mentioned earlier, the health care culture values autonomy and independence. Patients, on the other hand, often value the family over the individual, and prefer to make decisions as a group and to assist the patient in "self-care" functions the staff thinks the patient should do on his or her own. Furthermore, many prefer to have family members with them at all times, leading to chaos and loss of control from the perspective of the nurses.

The health care culture's value of *efficiency* often conflicts with patients' value of *modesty*. Many doctors and nurses find concern about keeping patients covered difficult when their primary focus is performing an appropriate procedure. The health care culture also values *self-control.* Many patients, however, come from cultures in which emotional expressiveness is the norm. This can lead to resentment toward such patients on the part of the staff.

Problems also result from a disparity between the world view of the health care culture and that of the patient population.

World View

The second most important concept for understanding people's behavior is to understand their world view. People's world view consists of their basic assumptions about the nature of reality. These become the foundation for all actions and interpretations. Religion largely defines the world view of people who are devoutly religious. Belief in the existence of God, for example, might be part of their world view. If people believe God confers both health and illness, it may be very difficult to get them to take certain medications or change their health behavior. They might not share the health care culture's belief that germs cause disease and that diet and exercise contribute to one's health. They would see no point worrying about high blood pressure or bacteria when moral behavior is the key to good health.

Since people's world view consists of their *assumptions* about the nature of reality, they rarely question the veracity of their beliefs. For example, would a devout Christian conclude that God does not exist on the basis of the accidental slaughter of innocent children? Probably not. Rather, the Christian might see it as further proof that "God works in mysterious ways." No matter how much "evidence" is presented to the contrary, people rarely change or even question their world view. Instead, they reinterpret events in a manner consistent with their beliefs.

Emic and Etic

The terms "emic" and "etic," derived from linguistics and rarely used in ordinary life, are extremely important in anthropology. They refer to perspectives. Emic perspectives are the insiders' perspectives, natives' views of their own behavior. Etic perspectives are those of outsiders. These two simply represent different vantage points, and knowing both helps provide a more complete picture, a fact which caregivers would do well to remember when treating patients from different cultures. Try to understand *their* perspective on their condition, as well as your own.

People's Relationship to Nature

Another aspect of world view involves people's relationship to nature. American culture, for example, believes people can control nature. If the land is dry, they irrigate. If the disease is caused by bacteria, they destroy the bacteria. If the heart does not work, they replace it. This also relates to the health care culture's view of the body as a machine; if it becomes broken, one should quietly turn it over to the mechanics (doctors and nurses) to be fixed. To the consternation of many health care professionals, not all cultures share that belief.

Other cultures, such as Asian and Native American, see people as a part of nature. They strive to maintain harmony with the earth, and look to the land to provide treatment for disease. Herbal remedies are important in their cultures. Still other cultures, such as Hispanic, believe people have little or no control over natural forces. *Que será, será.* Preventive health care measures are likely to be ignored. They would do no good anyway. What will be, will be. Thus world view can have important implications for health-related behavior.

Ethnocentrism and Cultural Relativism

Two key anthropological concepts are ethnocentrism and cultural relativism. They refer to attitudes. *Ethnocentrism* is the view that one's culture's way of doing things is the right and natural way. All other ways are inferior, unnatural, perhaps even barbaric. *Cultural relativism* is the attitude that other ways of doing things are different but equally valid. It tries to understand the behavior in its cultural context. Most humans are ethnocentric. It is natural to think one's own culture's way is best. Anthropologists, however, strive to be culturally relativistic.

If I were to tell most Americans about a group of people in Africa who sometimes kill healthy newborn infants, they would probably take the ethnocentric attitude that these people were barbarians. If I were to explain that they were hunters and gatherers living on the edge of starvation and that if a second child is born too close to the first, chances are about 100 percent that both will die because the mother does not have enough milk to support both, their attitude might change. They still might not condone infanticide, but they might understand it as the only viable choice in a desperate situation. Rather than seeing the Africans as barbarians, they might realize that the people were forced to extreme measures by hopeless circumstances. Their attitude would thus change from being ethnocentric to culturally relativistic.

The Western health care system tends to be ethnocentric because practitioners believe that their approaches to healing are superior to all others. There is a lot we can learn, however, from other cultures. Many modern drugs, including quinine, were derived from plants used by native peoples. Westerners are beginning to acknowledge the effectiveness of acupuncture for certain conditions. The goal of all systems of healing is the same—to help people get well. If all cultures could study each other's techniques with a culturally relativistic perspective, the cause of modern medicine would be greatly advanced.

Time Orientation

Time orientation, one's focus regarding time, varies in different cultures. No individual or culture will look exclusively to the past, present, or future, but most will tend to emphasize one over the others. Chinese, British, and Austrian cultures have a past orientation. They are traditional and believe in doing things the way they have always been done. Interestingly, in many cases, countries that emphasize the past are ones that were once more powerful than they are now. This may be their way of recognizing and valuing that time in their history. These cultures usually prefer traditional approaches to healing rather than accepting each new procedure or medication that comes out.

People with a predominantly present time orientation may also be less likely to utilize preventive health measures. They reason that there is no point taking a pill for hypertension when they feel fine, especially if the pill is expensive and inconveniently causes unpleasant side effects. They do not look ahead in hope of preventing a stroke or heart attack, or they may feel they will deal with it when it happens. Poverty often forces people into a present time orientation. They are not likely to make plans for the future when they are concerned with surviving today.

Middle-class white American culture tends to be future oriented. That is reflected in the medical system's stress on preventive medicine and enthusiasm for each new medical technique or drug. In contrast to past-oriented cultures, progress and change are highly valued. China is also shifting to a future orientation, as evidenced by the long-term plan to reduce the country's population by limiting family size.

Hispanics and African Americans tend to have a present time orientation. This does not mean that they do not recognize the past or the future, but living in the present is more important to them. Their concept of the future may also be different from the Anglo concept. For example, African Americans are more likely to say "I'll see you" than "I'll see you tomorrow." The former implies the future but is not specific. The future arrives in its own time. From this point of view, one cannot be late. Conflict may occur, however, in interactions with white middle-class people, for whom time is very specific.

As the last statement implies, time orientation can also refer to degree of adherence to clock time. From the perspective of one oriented to the clock, someone who arrives at 3:15 for a 2:30 appointment is late. For someone who does not focus on clock time, both represent mid-afternoon.

This type of time orientation appears to be related to subsistence economy. In countries with economies based on agriculture, people tend to be more relaxed about time; as I like to say, "The crops don't care what time they get picked." Many people in traditional agricultural villages do not own clocks; the pace is slower and more attuned to nature's rhythms. In contrast, industrialized nations must pay attention to clock time. There are large numbers of people to organize, and each must complete his or her task according to schedule in order for the next person to begin. Without clocks, chaos would reign.

Hierarchical Versus Egalitarian Cultures

Just as cultures differ in time orientation, they also vary in social structure. American culture is organized according to an egalitarian model. Theoretically, everyone is equal. Status and power are dependent on an individual's personal qualities rather than age, sex, family, occupation, or any other characteristic. In reality, things may operate differently, but we hold equality as our ideal. Some cultures such as Asian are based on a hierarchical model. Everyone is not equal. Status is based on such characteristics as age, sex, and occupation. Status differences are seen as important, and people of higher status command respect. Social structure, then, can have an important influence on the way people interact, as will be seen in many of the examples given later in this book.

Family of Orientation Versus Family of Procreation

During the course of their lives, many people are members of two different family groups—the family they are born into and the one they create through marriage and children. Anthropologists distinguish the two as "family of orientation" and "family of procreation." The family of orientation is the one a person is born into, the one to which one first orients oneself. It includes the individual, parents, brothers and sisters, and any other household members. The family of procreation is the one formed through marrying and procreating. It includes the individual, spouse, and children. Some cultures, particularly those in which the married couple continues to reside with the parents of the bride or groom, emphasize the family of orientation. Other cultures emphasize the family of procreation. Americans tend to set up their own nuclear family households, and that family takes precedence over all others. The result is a differing set of loyalties, as will be discussed in Chapter 6.

Disease Etiology

Most Americans believe that germs cause disease. Not all cultures share that belief, however. Other causes of disease include upset in body balance; soul loss, soul theft, and spirit possession; breach of taboo; and object intrusion. Treatment for diseases resulting from such etiologies must vary to be appropriate to the cause.

Upset in body balance is a notion that appears to have originated in China and spread from there to influence beliefs in Asia, India, Spain, and Latin America. It refers to the belief that a healthy body is in a state of balance. When it gets out of balance, illness results. In Asia, the balance is between *yin* and *yang*. All things in the universe are primarily either yin or yang, including diseases, which may result from excess yin, excess yang, deficient yin, or deficient yang. Yin and yang are generally translated as hot (yang) and cold (yin), although these refer to qualities, not temperatures. For example, we perceive chili peppers as hot, even if they have been refrigerated.

The balance between hot and cold can be upset by a number of factors, including an improper balance of foods and strong emotional states. The goal of treatment is to restore balance to the system. This is generally accomplished through the use of foods (for example, cold foods should be eaten to cure a hot illness), herbs, or other treatments. To prevent disease, one should avoid extremes, such as ice water. Diet is exceedingly important. (Dietary staples such as rice are generally thought to be neutral, a fortunate and practical designation.)

Foods that are hot in one culture may be cold in another, so it is difficult to make up a comprehensive list. Patients' beliefs in hot and cold qualities can generally be ascertained only by observing their behavior. If they refuse certain foods or medications, it may be that an illness they perceive as hot is being treated with a hot food or medication. Offering other foods or liquids to take with the pill to "neutralize" it may solve the problem. If they will not take the pill with ice water, they might take it with hot tea, orange juice, or hot chocolate.

Although the importance of maintaining a balance between hot and cold is not recognized in Western medicine, there is a growing recognition that stress plays an important role in affecting the immune system's ability to fight disease. Stress represents a kind of imbalance. Recent studies indicate that a person's emotional state may also have a significant influence on the immune system. Thus, though the words we use are different, body balance is a notion to which we should be able to relate.

Paradoxically, China is moving away from traditional medicine in favor of Western medicine, while there is increasing interest in the United States in traditional Chinese healing practices. When I asked several Chinese nurses how they integrate the concept of yin and yang with germ theory, they explained that when yin and yang are out of balance, germs can cause disease. This is nearly identical to the Western notion of the relationship between stress and disease.

Soul loss, along with related *soul theft,* is another category of disease etiology. The concept is self-explanatory. The soul has either left the body on its own or been stolen, leaving the body in a weakened and ill state. The goal of treatment is to return the soul to the body. It usually requires a specialist, such as a shaman, who can "leave" his or her own body to search for and return the missing soul. Although Western medicine lacks a similar etiological category, catatonic schizophrenics can be described metaphorically as bodies with "no one home."

Spirit possession involves the taking over of the victim's body by a spirit being. The victim usually acts in ways that are inappropriate for him or her. In some cultures, this may give the victim a form of power. It is generally the poor, the oppressed, and minorities who become "possessed." For example, in Ethiopia, women may become possessed by powerful "Zar" spirits. When this occurs, their husbands must treat them with unaccustomed kindness and respect, for they are no longer dealing with their wives but with powerful Zars. The negative side of possession by a Zar is that the woman is thought to be crazy and must seek help through a Zar cult. Exorcism is the treatment for spirit possession.

The next etiological category is *breach of taboo,* which means doing something forbidden, whether it is eating food cooked by a menstruating woman, speaking directly to one's mother-in-law, or, among some Christian sects, having extramarital or homosexual relations. Disease is the punishment meted out by a supernatural force such as God. Treatment involves penance and atonement.

The final major category is of *object intrusion.* It refers to the condition in which a magical foreign object enters the body and causes the individual to become ill. Treatment involves removing the object. In most cases, a shaman will suck it out from the afflicted part of the patient's body. The shaman then produces the offending object. Upon analysis, the object often turns out to be bits of hair, animal parts, teeth, or plant material, mixed with blood from the shaman's mouth. One shaman, accused by an anthropologist of practicing legerdemain, freely admitted to secreting the object in his mouth prior to sucking it out of the patient's body. He explained that the real object he removed was invisible, but that it was important for the patient to see something tangible, so he practiced a bit of sleight of hand (or mouth) for the patient's psychological benefit.

Two important points should be made regarding disease etiology. First, the treatment must be appropriate to the cause. If germs cause disease, kill the germs. If the body is out of balance, restore balance. If the soul is gone, retrieve it. If a spirit has taken over the body, exorcise it. If a rule has been violated, do penance. If an object has entered the body, remove it. All these remedies are perfectly logical. Whether these etiologies are the true causes of the disease is irrelevant. A patient who believes he or she is ill because of soul loss will not be cured by any amount of antibiotics. The mind is very powerful, as the placebo effect demonstrates. The patient's beliefs, as well as body, must be treated. Many Americans feel they have not been treated properly if they do not receive an antibiotic for a virus, even though antibiotics are effective only against bacteria. Psychologically, they need the pill to get well.

Second, we must not let our ethnocentrism blind us to the merits in the beliefs of other cultures. They may be right. It is easy to look down on other systems, citing science to support Western medical beliefs. But all medical systems are based on observed cause-and-effect relationships. The major difference with the scientific approach is that science is falsifiable. A scientific hypothesis can be proven wrong. The beliefs of other systems cannot.

At the level of the individual, however, Americans demand no more proof than do people of any other culture. Most believe germs cause disease because their mothers told them so. Few have ever actually seen a germ, and fewer demand to see proof of viruses or bacteria at work. The experts have done that, and their word, along with our mothers', is enough. The same is true in other cultures. People believe disease is caused by spirit possession or object intrusion because their mothers and cultural experts told them so. They have seen people become ill when that happens and get well when treated. What further proof is necessary?

Theoretical Perspective

As can be inferred from the preceding sections, the underlying theoretical perspective is based upon adaptation theory. I believe that, in most cases, people have developed traditions designed to achieve success in the broader environment in which they live. This includes adaptations to both the physical and social environment. Obviously, there are exceptions, and there are other theoretical approaches which are equally fruitful in explaining people's behavior. However, this is the theory that will inform the interpretations given in this book. When cultural conflicts occur, it is often because what is successful under one set of environmental circumstances may be less so under others.

Cultural Customs

Utilizing adaptation theory, it can be argued that most cultural practices originate for very practical reasons. People, however, do not always act in a practical manner if the benefit to them is not obvious and immediate. They may need a "higher" purpose. Ideological injunctions are much more likely to be followed, as anthropologist Marvin Harris, a leading proponent of the cultural materialism approach, points out.

For example, the Hindu prohibition against killing cows may seem bizarre in a country where most people are starving, but it has a practical basis. Most cows are malnourished and if slaughtered would provide very little food. Living, however, cows are good substitutes for tractors. Their milk provides food. Their dung provides fertilizer, fuel for cooking, and, mixed with water, an excellent household flooring material. Far more use is made of living cows than could ever be gained from dead ones. Hungry individuals, however, might look at a cow and see dinner. Forgetting the animal's other practical uses, they might kill and eat it. But if the animal is made sacred, religious ideology will prevent such killing.

Circumstances sometimes change, obliterating the practical need for a custom. Ideology, however, is enduring and soon becomes tradition. Although many cultural and religious traditions no longer have any practical value, they have an important psychological one—they provide a sense of identity and belonging. They serve as a strong reminder that the individual is not like everyone else; he or she belongs to a special group. Abstaining from meat when everyone else is having hamburgers reminds the Hindu that he is Hindu. Walking to temple instead of driving on the Sabbath reminds the Jew that she is Jewish. In fact, the more difficult or impractical the custom, the stronger the reminder of ethnic or religious identity. Thus the benefits of adhering to seemingly outmoded customs can be enormous in a country like the United States, where feelings of isolation and anomie may be strong.

Chapter 2
Communication and Time Orientation

Miscommunication is a frequent problem in hospitals. The most obvious case is when the patient and the hospital personnel do not speak the same language. Interpreters are not always available. When they are, vocabulary may be insufficient. But these problems are obvious. There are more subtle ones that result from cultural differences in verbal and non-verbal communication styles and patterns. This chapter will explore these problems in communication as well as another subtle but provocative source of difficulty—cultural differences in time orientation. Patients and staff members may operate on different "time clocks," causing confusion and resentment for all parties.

Idioms

6   Idioms or other nonliteral expressions can also create misunderstanding. A Chinese-born physician called the night nurse one evening to check on a patient scheduled for surgery the next day. The nurse advised the physician that she noticed a new hesitancy in the patient's attitude. "To tell you the truth, doctor, I think Mrs. Colby is getting cold feet." The physician was not familiar with this idiom, suspected circulation problems, and ordered vascular tests.

7   A nervous patient jokingly asked his surgeon if he were going to "kick the bucket." The Korean physician, wanting to reassure the patient that his upcoming surgery would be successful, responded affably, "Oh, yes, you are definitely going to kick the bucket!" The patient was not reassured.

Another English

Language problems can also occur among native English speakers. In England, South Africa, and Australia, the word "fanny" is a derogatory term referring to a woman's vagina. Imagine the shock and horror of a British woman—or the confusion of a British man—when told to prepare for a shot in the fanny. (A South African nurse was appalled when an American aerobics instructor called out to her class, "Tighten your fanny, shake your fanny!") Similarly, birth control instruction to speakers of the "Queen's English" could be confusing if the instructor referred to a condom as a "rubber." Erasers are not a very effective means of preventing pregnancy.

Same Language, Different Meaning

Words can have different meanings in the same language. In Mexico, the word "horita" means right now. In Puerto Rico, it means in an hour or so. This could cause confusion between two Spanish speakers. Similarly, "just now" in South Africa means "later" in America. A South African immigrant reported frequent problems with her boss. At times, when he asked her to do something, she would reply, "I'll get to it just now." He'd come back an hour later, asking for the work, which hadn't been done. He would be angry; she had said she would do it right away, but hadn't. She, on the other hand, would be upset because she told him she would get to it later, and now he was expecting her to have it done immediately.

Even American English can have different meanings for hearing and deaf people. While Kelly, a young gay male was a patient in the hospital, blood was drawn for an HIV test. When the results came back, no interpreters for the deaf were available. Since Kelly was adept at reading lips, he was given the test results directly. He was told that his results were positive, meaning, of course, that he was HIV-positive. In deaf culture, however, "positive" means good, "negative" means bad. Kelly was relieved to hear that his test results were "positive"; that meant he was *not* HIV-positive! He went home and did not return for follow-up. What the nurse should have done was tell him that the results came back negative—that he was, indeed, HIV-positive.

This incident was not unique. The nurse who reported this said that another nurse she met at a deaf conference reported the same situation with a different patient. When working with the deaf, it is important to realize that the same words may have different connotations. It is critical to make sure that you give enough explanation to ensure that the patient truly understands the information given. It is rather surprising that the person giving the test results did not read Kelly's nonverbal reaction; his misunderstanding of the results must surely have resulted in an inappropriate emotional response (such as relief).

Same Word, Different Language

9   Sometimes the same word can have different meanings in different languages. Consuela, a Filipino nurse, had for several days been caring for Ramon Ibañez, a premature Mexican baby in intensive care. Everything seemed fine, until the Ibañezes suddenly requested that another nurse be assigned to their baby. Consuela was shocked, particularly since they had not given the social worker any explanation.

Consuela had Graciela, a Spanish speaking co-worker, ask them to explain the problem. They were a bit hesitant, but finally told her that they had overheard Consuela talking to a co-worker and mentioning that she had a "puto." In Spanish, *puto* refers to a male prostitute. Their baby's health had gotten worse; they assumed it was because Consuela had picked up a disease from her male prostitute and passed it on to their child. They were in fact a bit surprised that the hospital would employ such a woman to care for the infants.

Was Consuelo really seeing a male prostitute? No. In the Philippines, a *puto* is a rice cake. Consuelo had been telling her co-worker that she was having a rice cake for lunch. Graciela explained this to the Ibañezes and clarified that babies born severely premature often got worse before getting better; Ramon's condition had nothing to do with Consuelo. Fortunately, they understood their misunderstanding. The next week, Consuelo brought the Ibañezes some *puto* to eat. Mrs. Ibañez hugged her and again expressed their apologies.

In Dutch, the word for shower is *douche*. In English, douche is related to personal feminine hygiene. A hospitalized American patient might be a bit disconcerted if her Dutch nurse told her it was time for a douche.

"Boy"

10   Certain words have negative and inflammatory associations when used by the wrong people. Lavelle, who is African American, was the primary nurse for four sixteen-year-old Black gang members. She had developed a good relationship with them and treated them like her own children. When one got out of line, she would simply say, "Boy, keep your mouth shut and go somewhere and sit down." They usually complied.

One day, Susan, an Anglo nurse, tried the same tactic with one of them. It was time for Earl to go to physical therapy, but he was giving Susan a hard time. She assumed from his smile that he was joking. Finally, she tried Lavelle's approach. "Come on, boy," she said. "I'm not kidding with you. You have to go to therapy."

Earl flew into a rage and started swearing at Susan. Lavelle had to help calm him down. Susan was confused. He had never responded that way to Lavelle. She had not considered that the term "boy" is inoffensive when used by one Black person speaking to another but is highly insulting when used by Caucasians because of its origins among slaveowners.

Colleen, an Anglo nurse from Canada, learned the meaning of "boy" the hard way. Her first job when she moved to the United States was at an inner city hospital. The cafeteria was crowded the first day she was there, but she found an empty place across from two Black men. She went over to them and asked very sweetly, "Do you boys mind if I sit down here?" One answered her by picking up his plate of food and throwing it at her.

11

Most people would agree that he overreacted, but his response is understandable in the context of race relations in this country. The misunderstanding occurred because Canada has not had the same racial problems as the United States, and in the part of the country Colleen was from, adult men and women commonly refer to each other as boys and girls. No insult is meant or taken. Once someone explained the reason for the man's reaction to Colleen, she did not make that mistake again.

Many people know that "boy" is highly insulting to a Black man, but few are aware that the term "gal" has similar connotations for many Black women. Black slave women were called "gals," which explains why several Anglo nurses reported receiving cold and hostile glares from African American nurses whom they innocently referred to as "gals."

First Names

African Americans' sensitivity to perceived slights to their dignity is not surprising given their history in this country. It is therefore especially important to show them respect. Mary Washington, an elderly Black woman, was in the recovery room after surgery. To assess her condition, Cheryl, her nurse, spoke her name, "Mary." The patient slowly opened her eyes and turned her head but made no further sign of acknowledgment. Cheryl became concerned because most patients responded readily and clearly at this point. Shortly afterward Cheryl called the woman Mrs. Washington. She then became alert, pleasant, and cooperative. She had perceived the use of her first name as a lack of respect .

12

Americans tend to refer to each other by their first names. It is considered a sign of friendliness and equality. To use a first name for anyone other than a close friend, however, is both inappropriate and discourteous in most cultures, including European. In nineteenth-century English novels, even teenage girls referred to each other as Miss ___ until they had been friends for at least a year. Hospital personnel should refer to all adult patients as Mr., Miss, Ms., or Mrs., unless instructed otherwise.

As a side note, all Egyptian names are essentially first names. The first one listed is yours, the second one is your father's, and the third is your grandfather's (even if you're female). Aziz Mohamad would properly be addressed as "Mr. Aziz" and his wife, Sheida, as "Mrs. Sheida," although in the United States, Mrs. Aziz would be acceptable.

With the Indochinese, the first name given is generally the family name, followed by the individual name. For example, Nguyen Thanh's family name is Nguyen, his given name is Thanh. When addressing him, use Mr. with his given name, "Mr. Thanh."

When "Yes" May Mean "No"

13   Cultural values can also create communication problems. Jackie, an Anglo nurse, was explaining the harmful side effects of the medication Adela Samillan, a Filipino patient, was to take at home after her discharge. Although Mrs. Samillan spoke some English, her husband, who was more fluent, served as interpreter. Throughout Jackie's explanation, the Samillans nodded in agreement and understanding and laughed nervously. When Jackie verbally tested them on the information, however, it was apparent that they understood very little. What had happened?

Dignity and self-esteem are important for all individuals, but particularly so for most Asians. Had the Samillans indicated that they did not understand Jackie's instructions, they would have lost their self-esteem for not understanding or they would have caused Jackie to lose hers for not explaining the material well enough. By pretending to understand, Mr. and Mrs. Samillan felt they were preserving everyone's dignity.

Jackie's first clue should have been their nervous laughter. Giggling is often a sign of discomfort and embarrassment. Once Jackie realized they had not understood the material, she went over it until they were able to explain it back to her. It is important not to take smiles and nods of agreement for understanding when dealing with Asian patients. They should be asked to demonstrate their understanding.

14   A second incident involved Linh Lee, a sixty-four-year-old Chinese woman hospitalized for an acute evolving heart attack. At discharge, her physician suggested that she come back in two weeks for a follow-up examination. She agreed to do so, but never returned. It is likely that she never intended to do so but agreed because he was an authority figure. Chinese are taught to value accommodation. Rather than refuse to the physician's face and cause him dishonor, Mrs. Lee agreed. She simply did not follow through, sparing everyone embarrassment.

Grammar

The cases described above involved the use of the word "yes" to avoid the embarrassment of saying "no." There is another occasion in which "yes" may be used inappropriately (from the American perspective) for reasons of grammar. According to common English usage, if someone were asked, "Haven't you taken your medication yet today?" and they had not taken it, they would answer, "No." According to the rules of grammar found in most Asian languages, the accurate response would be "Yes," as in "Yes, it is a true statement that I have not yet taken my medication today." The English speaker would be misled by the Asian patient's affirmative response, thinking that person had already taken the medication when he or she had not. To reduce possible confusion, it is generally best to avoid sentences with negatives.

A related source of misunderstanding involves the phrase, "Would you mind . . ." If you ask an Asian, "Would you mind . . . ?" you will probably receive the answer "yes." Americans would generally interpret that to mean the other individual does mind, but they would be wrong. It is the Asian way of showing agreement or willingness.

Pronouns

Different languages have characteristics that are not directly translatable, as anyone who has struggled with the task of remembering the gender of inanimate objects in French or Spanish knows well. English poses a similar problem for many Asians. Mieko, a Japanese nurse, was assigned to care for six patients, two male and four female. During report, she consistently referred to the female patients as "he." Her supervisor interrupted to point out that there were no male patients in the bed numbers she mentioned. Mieko acknowledged that fact and continued in the same manner. The supervisor became confused. Had four transsexuals slipped in?

The explanation is simple. Many Asian languages lack pronouns that reflect gender; "he" and "she" do not exist. Thus Asians have no model for using the pronouns "he" or "she" and often mix them up, confusing everyone else in the process. This may seem surprising, given the importance of gender in Asian hierarchical cultures. It might help to think of it in this way—gender is of such importance that it is not diminished by the use of a mere pronoun. An individual would be referred to as "that man" or "that woman." Knowledge of this characteristic of the language can lessen the confusion.

The Use of Interpreters

Because there are many immigrants from a variety of linguistic backgrounds living in the United States, translation is often a problem within the hospital. Most hospitals lack the resources to maintain sufficient professional, staff interpreters to cover all the languages of the patient population. Often, family members are called upon to translate. This may be fine in some instances, but there are times when cultural elements interfere with proper interpretation.

16   An Hispanic woman, Graciela Mendoza, had to sign an informed consent form for a hysterectomy. Her bilingual son served as the interpreter. When he described the procedure to his mother, he appeared to be translating accurately and indicating the appropriate body parts. His mother signed willingly. The next day, however, when she learned that her uterus had been removed and that she could no longer bear children, she became very angry and threatened to sue the hospital. What went wrong?

Because it is inappropriate for an Hispanic male to discuss her private parts with his mother, the embarrassed son explained that a tumor would be removed from her abdomen and pointed to that general area. When Mrs. Garcia learned that her uterus had been removed, she was quite angry and upset because an Hispanic woman's status is derived in large part from the number of children she produces. When dealing with anything remotely sexual, it is best not to use family members; if necessary, at least make every effort to use same-sex family members. However, as the next case illustrates, this may not be sufficient.

17   An Arab woman had just given birth. Her Arab American mother-in-law was asked to translate the health teaching material to the new mother. All went well until the nurse reached the information on contraception. The mother-in-law refused to translate such information. She was part of a culture that valued large families, and she wanted as many grandchildren as possible.

In this case, the woman openly refused to translate. It is just as likely that she might have pretended to convey the information while actually talking about something else. It is important to remember that language is not the only issue involved in translation.

18   The next case occurred outside the hospital, as part of home health care. Tran Nyguen, a sixty-five-year old Vietnamese refugee, was living in a two-bedroom apartment of a resettlement camp with eight members of her extended family. They had all arrived in the United States two years earlier, so they still manifested their traditional customs. She had recently been discharged from an acute care hospital; she was suffering from lung cancer, along with tubercular cavitary lesions in the lungs.

Since Mrs. Nyguen did not speak English, her teenage granddaughter acted as interpreter. That this was a problem, however, was revealed by the fact that both the patient and the granddaughter would look at the eighty-year old uncle before speaking. He was the patriarch of the family and an important figure in this male dominant, hierarchical culture. Martha, the home health nurse, resolved the issue quite cleverly by having the granddaughter tell her uncle what the nurse wanted to say, and then the grandfather told the patient. When the patient responded, she would talk to the uncle who would then pass on the response to the granddaughter, who then translated for the nurse. While somewhat cumbersome, this method upheld the hierarchy within the Vietnamese family.

Taking a History

Nurses may sometimes experience difficulty when trying to obtain information from a patient. Jeanie did when trying to get a health history from a young Gypsy woman. The patient's mother-in-law insisted upon accompanying her to the examining room. Jeanie assumed she wanted to act as an interpreter, but her English skills were no better than her daughter-in-law's. The patient's reply to every question was the same: "I don't know." She probably knew many of the answers but was respecting a cultural prohibition against giving too much information to Gaje (non-Gypsies). The patient's mother-in-law may have been there in part to protect her and in part to make sure she did not reveal too much. [19]

Another situation involved a twenty-five-year-old Laotian refugee named Thongsouk Vongkhamkaew, who was being treated for stomach cancer. Although her English was proficient, she did not appear to have a full understanding of her disease and the treatments and life changes necessary for coping with it. Greg, a staff social worker, decided to arrange for a translator. When the nurse introduced Greg to Thongsouk so he could explain his plan, she appeared very nervous. She would not talk with him except to repeat, "Everything is okay." [20]

Thongsouk's fear and refusal to talk stemmed from her mistaken belief that Greg was with the military or government. After many decades of war, Laotians tend to distrust strangers. The patient might have feared that anything she said would have repercussions for her family still in Laos and Thailand. She did not understand the role of the social worker. There is no equivalent in Laos, where family and friends provide assistance and support, and hospitals are for medicine. She might have responded better if one of the doctors or nurses, whose role she understood and accepted, had talked with her instead.

Ramona was trying to get a medical history from Mrs. Cata, a Navaho [21] woman. After each question Ramona asked, there would be a long silence. When Ramona spoke, Mrs. Cata would often stare at the floor. Ramona assumed it meant that Mrs. Cata was shy and had trouble understanding her, but that was not the case. She was merely indicating in a culturally appropriate manner that she was paying close attention to Ramona. The Navaho value silence. A person who interrupts while someone is speaking is perceived as immature.

Most Americans are uncomfortable with silences and tend to fill them with words, making small talk. The Navaho use silence to formulate their thoughts. Words should have significance. An anthropologist doing fieldwork among the Navaho commented that it took her a long time to get used to talking with them. She would ask a question and get no response. She assumed they had not heard or understood her. She was wrong. They were trying to give her the most complete answer possible, and that took consideration. Eventually, she became comfortable with long pauses in conversation.

When dealing with Navaho patients, if they seem slow to respond, be patient. Give them time to consider your question before answering. Don't make judgments based upon the meaning of your own behavior.

Informed Consent

22   Mr. Fanous was a sixty-five-year old man from the Middle East who had come to the cardiac cath lab for a heart catheterization. It was Nina's job to get him to sign an informed consent. He read the form, which described the various complications that could result along with the pros and cons of the procedure. After Nina went through everything with him, he did not want to sign the form. He questioned why it was even necessary—why didn't they just go ahead and do the procedure? She explained to him that it was not ethical to talk someone into a procedure, but that it could not be done without his consent. After some discussion, Mr. Fanous finally signed the consent form.

Why had he been so reluctant to sign? Partly, it may have been because he did not want to be at the hospital in the first place; he had only come due to the urging of friends. From a cultural perspective, however, it may be because many Arabs believe that since the doctor is the one with the knowledge and training, the doctor should be the one to make the decision. What did Mr. Fanous know about heart catheterization? Why was the hospital so unwilling to take responsibility for their actions? Although as Nina suggests, there is probably no way to avoid this kind of cultural misunderstanding, just knowing what to expect might help the nurse.

Communication Styles and Demeanor

A twenty-seven-year-old Mexican American named Alfredo Gomez was   23
in traction with multiple fractures following a car accident. He whined
continuously and incessantly summoned Helga, his German nurse, with
the call light. Helga became very frustrated and angry with him and
consequently adopted a stern and direct attitude. Alfredo's behavior
changed only when his wife and sister arrived and gave him their full
attention. They anticipated his every need, straightening his pillow and
moistening his lips. Following their lead, Helga spoke more slowly and
warmly to Alfredo, letting him know she understood what a frightening
experience he had had. She also did what she could to make him more
comfortable before he asked. As a result, he quickly became less dependent and did not use the call light so frequently.

Why did Helga's change in behavior have this positive effect on him?
Helga had been raised to be strong and stoic when ill and thus had little
tolerance for Alfredo's whining and demanding behavior. She treated
him unemotionally, in the proper German manner. Mexicans, in contrast, are far more emotionally expressive. They expect to be pampered
when ill; it is one way the family shows love and concern. Alfredo was
feeling alone, frightened, and unloved because he was not receiving the
care and attention he expected. He became even more needy. Once he
was treated the way he expected to be, his anxiety and thus his neediness
were lessened.

Another difficult patient was a twenty-five-year-old upper-class Iranian   24
named Hamid Sadeghi. He was very uncooperative and refused to do
anything for himself. He would ring for the nurses and demand, "You
get here right now and do this." He would not, however, accept anything
he had not specifically requested, including lunch trays and medication.
He posted a sign on his door that read, "Do not enter without knocking,
including the nurses." His attitude caused a great deal of resentment
among the nurses. Why did he treat them this way?

When asked, Hamid responded, "This is the way it is done." Finally,
one of the nurses who had an Iranian brother-in-law recognized the behavior and explained. Traditionally, Iranian men are dominant over
Iranian women. They *give* orders to women, not take them. Furthermore,
as a member of the upper class, Hamid was probably used to giving orders to servants. He was not purposely being difficult but merely acting
in his customary manner.

Nursing is a low-level position in the Middle East because the job requires a woman to violate the laws of the Koran—she must both look at
and touch the bodies of naked male strangers. The Koran stipulates ex-

treme sexual segregation, primarily to protect the purity of women. Middle Eastern men may thus have little respect for the female nurse who trespasses their sacred laws in the performance of her duties. It is no wonder that Saudi Arabians pay huge salaries to foreign nurses; it is difficult to attract many Saudi women to the profession.

There was no happy resolution to Hamid's situation. Some of the nurses complied with his demands, some refused to care for him. All resented him. Once the nurses understood the reason for his behavior, they tried to discuss it with him. Their efforts went unrewarded, however, because Hamid was unwilling to accept American culture and they were unwilling to adapt themselves to his. The doctor tried to intervene, but Hamid would not budge. "I will treat the nurses as women should be treated," he maintained.

The nurses eventually pressured the doctor to discharge the patient because no one wanted to care for him. The doctor felt an early discharge would not endanger him, and Hamid was quite willing to leave. The incident did nothing to promote cross-cultural communication. Hamid's behavior toward the nurses was extreme, but it was based on Middle Eastern sex roles. A better solution would have been to assign a male nurse to his case.

Eye Contact

25

Ellen was trying to teach her Navaho patient, Jim Nez, how to live with his newly diagnosed diabetes. She soon became extremely frustrated because she felt she was not getting through to him. He asked very few questions and never met her eyes. She reasoned from this that he was uninterested and therefore not listening to her.

Rather than signaling disinterest, however, Mr. Nez's behavior demonstrated a respect for the nurse's authority. Mr. Nez's lack of eye contact probably reflected the Navaho belief that the eyes are the window to the soul. To make direct eye contact is disrespectful and can endanger the spirits of both parties. Thus his lack of eye contact actually displayed his concern.

A former student said she automatically rejected job applicants who did not make eye contact on the basis that they could not be trusted. In fact, there may be good cultural reasons why eye contact is purposely avoided.

Many Asians consider it disrespectful to look someone directly in the eye, especially if that person is in a superior position. Most Asian cultures are hierarchical; men are considered superior to women, parents to children, teachers to students, doctors to nurses, and so forth. Looking someone directly in the eye implies equality. An Asian patient may avoid eye contact out of respect for the "superior status" of the doctor or nurse, rather than for reasons of disinterest or dishonesty. A Korean nurse shared that when she scolded her children, she would get angry if they had the nerve to look her in the eye. She instructed them to show respect by looking down.

Many Middle Easterners regard direct eye contact between a man and a woman as a sexual invitation. Female doctors or nurses dealing with Middle Eastern men must be aware that their eye contact may be interpreted not as directness but as an invitation of a sexual nature. In general, eye contact should be avoided with Middle Easterners of the opposite sex. Medical personnel should be aware of the meaning of eye contact in their patients' culture and make sure the appropriate communication is both transmitted and received.

Touching

It is considered very poor taste in most Asian countries for people to touch in public. Men and women should not hug, kiss, or hold hands. It is, however, common for individuals of the same sex to hold hands or walk arm-in-arm. It merely indicates that they are close friends or relatives.

Juen, a former student from mainland China, told me that when she first came to the United States she was staying in the home of an American family. One evening, a male friend of the family came to visit. When he left, he lightly kissed everyone good-bye, including Juen. She was completely shocked, and said, "When he kissed me, it made me feel so uncomfortable, just like you ate a fly!"   26

Health care workers should be advised that many Asian co-workers and patients will not be comfortable with the casual touching and hugging that many Latinos and Americans do without even thinking. Observe their behavior (and that of their families) to see what they are comfortable with.

In class, one of my students asked me if I knew why the Orthodox   27
Jewish husband of one of her patients refused to shake her hand when she held it out to him. At the time, she thought he was being rude. He wasn't; he was merely following the Jewish prohibition against touching between members of the opposite sex. The same rule holds true for Muslims. Whenever possible, same-sex caregivers should be assigned to Orthodox Jews and Muslims, and opposite-sex touching should be avoided.

Gestures

Nonverbal communication can be equally problematical. An Anglo patient named Jon Smith called out to Maria, a Filipino nurse: "Nurse,   28 nurse." Maria came to Mr. Smith's door and politely asked, "May I help you?" Mr. Smith beckoned for her to come closer by motioning with his right index finger. Maria remained where she was and responded in an angry voice, "What do you want?"

Mr. Smith was confused. Why had Maria's manner suddenly changed? The problem was that the innocent "come here" gesture is used in the Philippines (and in Korea) only to call animals, and in a sense Mr. Smith had called Maria a dog. To summon a person, Filipinos motion with the whole hand, palm in, fingers down.

29   Unfortunately, many Americans are confused as to whether this gesture means "come here" or "go away," as Teresa, a Filipino nurse, discovered when she tried to call Nancy, a nurse's aide, to assist her with a patient. She motioned to her, palm in, fingers down, to come over. Rather than move nearer to Teresa, Nancy merely smiled and waved back, using the same gesture. At the time, Teresa was confused and a bit hurt over Nancy's refusal to help her. She later learned that Nancy simply thought she was waving good-bye.

Problems such as this can best be handled through in-service education classes. If hospital personnel from other cultures are taught the different meanings of gestures, they might not take offense. Maria might have responded to Mr. Smith's request and then politely explained how she felt about the gesture. Mr. Smith would have learned something important about cross-cultural communication and probably refrained from using that gesture with a Filipino again.

Other seemingly innocuous gestures that can create misunderstandings include the "okay" sign (thumb and index fingers together in a circle, other fingers straight up), the "thumbs-up" sign, and the "V" made with the index and middle fingers (used to signify either peace or victory). In Brazil, the "okay" sign is a crude sexual invitation. "Thumbs-up" in Iran and the "V," held palm in, in South Africa are insulting gestures similar to the raised middle finger in U.S. culture.

Time Orientation

30   Matilda Rojas was a fifty-six-year-old first generation Mexican American woman with an incarcinated hernia. She was referred to a local home IV infusion company on discharge, and an appointment was made for the pharmacist and IV specialist nurse to meet with Mrs. Rojas's family in the patient's hospital room. The discharge planner arranged the appointment for "lunchtime."

The pharmacist and nurse arrived at Mrs. Rojas's room exactly at noon. They had to wait for the Rojas family over an hour. The first misunderstanding was over the meaning of "lunchtime." For the Rojas family, it meant between one and two P.M., not twelve o'clock. They made no apology for their lateness, since they thought they were on time. The pharmacist and nurse, both rushed for time with appointments scheduled throughout the day, were rather upset. They saw the Rojases as uneducated, low-class Mexican Americans with little consideration or respect for others. While they did not say anything to the family, they were impatient and irritable with them. Sensing their irritation, the Rojases became quiet and withdrawn, not participating in the patient's care. The session was a waste, since it is impossible to do home IV care instruction without the cooperation of both the patient and the family. The pharmacist and nurse told the discharge planner that the patient and family were untrainable, and thus inappropriate for home IV therapy.

The problems began when the discharge planner made the appointment in relation to an activity (lunch) rather than at a set time. Not every culture eats meals at the same time. In many European countries, for example, it is common to eat dinner at ten o'clock in the evening. Americans tend to see time in discrete units, each needing to be filled. The pharmacist and nurse had scheduled several appointments throughout the day; a delay in one created havoc with their entire schedule. The Rojases, on the other hand, were not as bound to the clock. Hispanics tend to see time more expansively and to be more present oriented. There is more focus on the present activity than on future ones.

If you need to schedule an appointment with someone who has a different time orientation from you, make sure that you specify clock time, with the explanation that you have another appointment at a specific time and will have to leave if the other person is excessively late.

Another incident featuring a conflict in time orientation involved Ikem Nwoye, a Nigerian nurse assistant. He would come to the hospital, clock in, and then go to the lounge to have a cigarette and chat. The nurses were often waiting with patients who were signed out and ready to be transferred to Ikem's room. His lack of concern for punctuality created a hardship for the other nurses. They thought he should be fired. They had many difficulties with him, including his inability to take orders from women (which will be discussed in Chapter 8). In such cases, when numerous discussions of the problem fail to resolve it, termination may be the only answer.

31

I once had an experience with a Native American woman involving present time orientation. I had bought some pottery from her on a trip through the Southwest. A friend admired one of the pots so I decided to try to get her one as a combination Christmas and house-warming present. I had a photograph of the artist holding the pot, which I sent, along with a letter, to the tourist center in her village. I asked if she could make

32

an identical pot for me and, if so, the cost. I gave her my phone number and enclosed a self-addressed stamped envelope.

Two months passed. I assumed that the letter had never reached her. Then, late on a Monday afternoon, I got a phone call from her. She was in town for an Indian art show that had been held that weekend. She had made the pot for me and asked if I wanted to pick it up now. She was leaving the city early the next morning.

She was staying on the other side of town, and it was rush hour. I arranged to meet her in the parking lot of a mall later that evening, when the traffic died down. I bought the pot, and my friend loved it. It struck me, however, that I had experienced a wonderful, if frustrating, example of present time orientation. The potter might have called or written to let me know she was coming to town. Instead, she waited until the very last moment to call me and make arrangements. She was operating with a present time orientation. She dealt with things when they needed to be done, not before. Many Indian languages, in fact, have no word for time.

As mentioned in Chapter 1, Third World cultures often have a present time orientation. Their economies are usually based on agriculture and thus do not require adherence to a clock, an object many people may not even own. It is only in industrialized nations that clock time is important because the performance of everyone's job depends on all others doing theirs. It becomes necessary to adhere to a standard of time.

Health care professionals can do little about the present time orientation of patients. It is difficult for people who are not used to running their lives by the clock, who think it is rude to interrupt one activity to start another, and whose poverty makes it difficult for them to adhere to other people's schedules to change their ways. The best health care professionals can do is to stress how important it is that patients show up on time for scheduled appointments. But they should be prepared for patients to be late.

When one is dealing with co-workers who operate with a present time orientation, more drastic measures may have to be taken. One person's tardiness can be hard on the rest of the staff and on the patients. If after several discussions and warnings, a tardy staff member does not change, he or she may have to be fired. It is important, however, that everyone realizes that the tardiness is a cultural trait, not a defect in the person's character.

Summary

Miscommunication between health care professionals and their patients often has nothing to do with ethnic background. A common problem is the use of medical jargon, for example, "voided" instead of "peed." Patients may lack the technical vocabulary to describe their symptoms in a way that physicians can understand. Some patients may be very forth-right, whereas others may need probing; a health care provider must be sensitive to different communication styles. Patients may be too embar-rassed to discuss certain problems, particularly those of a sexual nature. A health care provider needs excellent communication skills to be able to handle sensitive issues.

When the health care provider and the patient are of different ethnic backgrounds, there are numerous additional opportunities for misunder-standings. Communication styles and time orientation vary considerably from culture to culture, causing confusion and sometimes annoyance for hospital personnel. As a further complication, people from different cul-tures may behave in similar ways but for different reasons. Understand-ing why people communicate (or do not) in the way they do, however, can help relieve the frustration of health care workers and perhaps con-tribute to better patient care.

For additional issues related to informed consent, see Chapters 6 and 7.
For additional issues related to language and communication, see Chapter 8.

Chapter 3
Pain

An important health care issue is the treatment of pain. Before it can be treated, however, it must be properly assessed. This can cause confusion for health care providers who are unaware of cultural differences in response to pain, particularly in how it is expressed. Also critical are cultural variations in attitudes toward the use of pain medication.

Expression of Pain

33   Differing responses to pain are well illustrated in the cases of Mr. Wu and Mr. Valdez. Bobbie, the nurse, had two patients who had both had coronary artery by-pass grafts. Mr. Valdez, a middle-aged Nicaraguan gentleman, was the first to come up from the recovery room. He was already hooked up to a morphine PCA (patient-controlled analgesia) machine, which allowed him to administer pain medication as needed in controlled doses and at controlled intervals. For the next two hours, he summoned Bobbie every ten minutes to request more pain medication. Bobbie finally called the physician to have his dosage increased and to request additional pain injections every three hours as needed. Every three hours he requested an injection. He continually whimpered in painful agony.

    Mr. Wu, a Chinese patient, was transferred from the recovery room an hour later. In contrast to Mr. Valdez, he was quiet and passive. He, too, was in pain, since he used his PCA machine frequently, but he did not show it. When Bobbie offered supplemental pain pills, he refused them. Not once did he use the call light to summon her.

    This is an instance of two patients with the same condition, yet vastly different ways of handling the pain. Nurses usually report that "expressive" patients often come from Hispanic, Middle Eastern, and Mediterranean backgrounds, while "stoic" patients often come from Northern European and Asian backgrounds. However, simply knowing a person's

ethnicity will not allow you to predict accurately how a patient will respond to pain, and, in fact, there are great dangers in stereotyping, as
the next case demonstrates.

Mrs. Mendez, a sixty-two-year-old Mexican patient, had just had a
femoral-popliteal by-pass graft on her right leg. She was still under se-
dation when she entered the recovery room, but an hour later, she
awoke and began screaming, "*Aye! Aye! Aye! Mucho dolor!* (much pain)."
Robert, her nurse, immediately administered the dosage of morphine
the doctor had prescribed. This, however, did nothing to diminish
Mrs. Mendez's cries of pain. He then checked her vital signs and pulse;
all were stable. Her dressing had minimal bloody drainage. To all ap-
pearances, Mrs. Mendez was in good condition. Robert soon became angry over her outbursts and stereotyped her as a "whining Mexican female
who, as usual, was exaggerating her pain."

After another hour, Robert called the physician. The surgical team
came on rounds and opened Mrs. Mendez's dressing. Despite a slight
swelling in her leg, there was minimal bleeding. However, when the physician inserted a large needle into the incision site, he removed a large
amount of blood. The blood had put pressure on the nerves and tissues
in the area and caused her excruciating pain.

She was taken back to the operating room. This time, when she returned and awoke in recovery, she was calm and cooperative. She complained only of minimal pain. Had the physician not examined her again
and discovered the blood in the incision site, Mrs. Mendez would have
probably suffered severe complications.

Despite the fact that Mexicans are generally expressive of their pain,
it does not mean that every Mexican patient will be, or that there is not
a legitimate basis for their cries. The generalizations in this chapter
(and book) are meant to be only generalizations; beware the dangers
of stereotyping—it can have disastrous consequences.

One case involving cultural differences in expressing pain had a tragic
ending. The Irish mother-in-law of one of my nursing students was in the
hospital. She was scheduled for surgery at the end of the week. Her
family became very concerned when she suddenly started complaining
of pain. They knew Mrs. Carroll was typically Irish in her stoicism. They
spoke to her doctor, who was from India. He was not worried. In his
country, women were usually vocal when in pain. He ignored their requests that the surgery be done sooner, thinking it unnecessary.

When he finally did operate, he discovered that Mrs. Carroll's condition had progressed to the point that she could not be saved. It is possible that if he had recognized her expressions of pain as a sign that
something was very wrong and had operated sooner, she might have
lived.

David Stein, a twenty-two-year-old Jewish patient suffering from fractured ribs following an auto accident, was both demanding and expressive. He made no effort to do anything for himself. David continually pushed the call light to have someone come straighten his covers or hand him the urinal, even though it was within easy reach. He brushed his teeth only when June, his nurse, steadfastly insisted. When he was turned over, stuck for lab work, or had his intravenous line restarted, he screamed so loudly that June was afraid people would think he was being tortured. When his mother came to visit, she hovered over him and acted solicitous.

A classic study done in a New York hospital in the early 1950s sheds some light on David's behavior. Mark Zborowski's project focused on three groups: Jews, Italians, and "Old Americans" (WASPs). These groups were selected because Jews and Italians had a reputation for exaggerating their pain, whereas the behavior of Old Americans was consistent with the values of the medical system; they were stoic and undemanding.

Although Jews and Italians reacted similarly to pain—loudly—they did so for different reasons. The Italians complained because the pain hurt. Pain medication usually satisfied them. This remedy was rarely effective with Jewish patients, however. In addition to everything else, they would then worry about becoming addicted. Their primary concern was not the pain sensation but the meaning and significance of the pain. How would it affect them and their families?

Zborowski observed that Jews and Italians have a similar socialization process. Children are warned to avoid injury, colds, and fights. Crying elicits sympathy, concern, and aid. The more they complain, the more attention and sympathy they receive. In many Jewish families, even a sneeze is seen as illness, thus predisposing children to become anxious about the meaning and significance of any symptoms. Jewish and Italian children are praised for avoiding physical injury and reprimanded for ignoring bad weather or drafts, or for playing rough games. Although this may not be as true today as it was at the time of the study, the behavior of older patients may still reflect this upbringing.

In contrast, Old American children are encouraged to participate in sports. Boys are taught to "take pain like a man" rather than "cry like a sissy" when injured. The body is seen as a machine, which, when not working (that is, when ill or injured) should be taken to a specialist (a doctor) and treated with as little fuss as possible.

Given their upbringings, it should not be surprising that adult Jews and Italians complain and desire attention when ill, while WASPs tend to be "easy" patients. When they are ill, most people revert to childhood behavior, even if the desired results are not forthcoming. If, like the Jewish patient described earlier, they were rewarded for complaining as children, they will complain as adults. If they were taught to lie quietly and not make a fuss, they will probably do the same when they grow up.

Most nurses find it difficult to care for patients like David, whose behavior was an extreme version of his culture. Nurses expect stoicism and compliance and do not get it. They thus tend to do as little as possible, and a new nurse is assigned to such patients each day. There are no easy solutions; extreme patience and understanding are required.

In contrast, some patients tolerate even the most severe pain with little   37
more than a clenched jaw and frequently will refuse pain medication. Osito Seisay, a Nigerian farmer who had been injured by a charging bull, was in the United States for arthro-microscopic knee surgery. His nurse waited for him to request pain medication, but he never did. Mr. Seisay was Muslim, and he offered his pain to Allah in thanks for the good fortune of being allowed such specialized surgery.

Why are people from some cultures generally more expressive of pain than those from others? One theory I would offer is that it has to do in part with the weather and degree of crowding. If it is cold, or heavily populated, such that large numbers of people are forced into close contact for long periods of time, it is generally advantageous to have people control their emotions. Otherwise, fights and general chaos are likely to result. In such cultures, such as those in northern Europe (cold weather) and Japan (crowding), individuals are socialized to control their emotions. The British, for example, take pride in having a "stiff upper lip." In warmer and less crowded conditions, if there is conflict, people can leave the scene. There is less inherent danger of chaos and, thus, no cultural "selection" for controlling one's emotions.

Requesting Pain Medication

Vickie, a research nurse dispensing experimental analgesics, noted that   38
an elderly Filipino patient named Fernando Abatay had not received any pain medication following his shoulder repair. When she asked him how much pain he was experiencing, he replied, "A lot." Vickie then questioned why he had not taken any medication. Mr. Abatay explained, "No one asked me if I wanted a shot and I didn't want to bother the nurses." The regular nurses assigned to him claimed that they could not tell he was in pain, and because he did not request any pain medication, they saw no need to give him any.

Mr. Abatay's behavior can be explained in part by the Filipino concept of *Bahala na* (God's will). Filipinos may appear stoic because they believe pain is the will of God and thus God will give them the strength to bear it. Besides, one cannot change it. This attitude is reminiscent of the fatalistic Hispanic concept *Que será, será.* A second explanation relates to Filipinos' respect for authority. Mr. Abatay did not want to bother the nurses. A professional's time is valuable, and unless one's problem is very serious, it is better left unmentioned.

39   Similarly, a middle-aged Chinese patient named Patrick Chang refused pain medication following cataract surgery. When asked, he replied that his discomfort was bearable and he could survive without any medication. Later, however, the nurse found him restless and uncomfortable. Again, she offered pain medication. Again he refused, explaining that her responsibilities at the hospital were far more important than his immediate comfort and he did not want to impose on her. Only after she firmly insisted that a patient's comfort was one of her most important responsibilities did Mr. Chang finally agree to take the medication.

His attitude is very different from that of most American patients. The Chinese, however, are taught self-restraint. Assertive and individualistic people are considered crude and poorly socialized. The needs of the group are more important than those of the individual. Inconspicuousness is highly valued and in recent history has proved necessary for survival. It is best not to call attention to oneself.

One other factor that may be involved in Asians' refusal of pain medication is courtesy. They generally consider it impolite to accept something the first time it is offered. Several nurses from mainland China said they often went hungry during the first few weeks of their stay in the United States. Whenever someone asked them if they wanted something to eat, they politely refused, awaiting a second offer. It rarely came. They soon learned that in America, if one does not accept something the first time, there may be no second chance. Hospital nurses are so busy that they seldom offer something more than once. They should be aware of Asian rules of etiquette when offering pain medication, food, back rubs, or other services.

The safest approach for the health care professional is to anticipate the needs of an Asian patient for pain medication without waiting for requests. If patients are told that their doctor ordered the medication, they will be less likely to refuse on the grounds of courtesy. Asians tend to respect the authority of the physician. But if patients continue to refuse medication, their wishes should be respected.

Attitudes Toward Pain Medication

40   Cecilia was a Filipino nurse in one of my classes. One day we were discussing the tendency of Filipino nurses to undermedicate their pain patients. If the physician prescribes a range of dosages, they will often administer the lowest dose. When asked about this, Filipino students

have given a number of explanations: pain medication is scarce in the Philippines, so they are trained not to use too much; addiction is highly feared; stoicism is valued; and, for Catholic Filipinos, there is virtue in suffering. After a few minutes, I noticed tears falling from Cecilia's eyes. When I asked her what was wrong, she explained that a year earlier her mother had died of cancer. The doctor had prescribed high dosages of pain medication in the months before her death. Cecilia administered the medication to her mother, but out of habit had cut each dosage in half before giving it to her mother. She did not want her mother to become addicted, she explained. Now, in class, she realized that she had allowed her mother to suffer needlessly. She was dying; what would it matter if she became addicted to the medication? The important lesson here is that caregivers must examine their own attitudes toward the use of pain medication and not let them affect the way they administer it to patients.

Filipinos are not the only group that tends to reject pain medication out of fear of addiction. Many East Indians share a similar attitude. Kari, a nurse from India, recounted the story of her aunt who recently had a total knee replacement. She went to visit her two days after she was discharged from the hospital. Kari noticed that her aunt seemed very tense. She asked her when she had last taken her pain medication. Before her aunt could answer, her son, a physician, responded, "Oh, Mom had her last pain medicine yesterday and she really does not need any more medicine. After all, we don't want her to get to used to taking the pain medication." In this case, reducing the pain medication had a negative impact on her aunt's health. She had stopped using her passive range-of-motion machine because it was too painful. By doing so, she risked not regaining full movement in her knee. It was important that her aunt take her pain medication as prescribed so she could become more mobile as well as more comfortable.

41

The potential problem might have been avoided if the health care provider had explained the rationale behind the use of pain medication. It's not merely to reduce the pain but also to allow her to do the rehabilitation exercises necessary for recovery.

Shots or Pills?

Mr. Hassan was an eighty-one-year-old Egyptian patient suffering from advanced lung cancer with bone metastases. Pain control was achieved with a long acting oral morphine. He was receiving hospice care from a home health agency. According to the hospital discharge planner, his pain was well controlled with two narcotic analgesic tablets twice a day; however, when the hospice nurse did her initial evaluation, she found

42

that the patient was requesting intramuscular or intravenous medications, despite the absence of pain between dosages. She explained to him that oral medications were preferable, but he was not satisfied. Two days later, he was readmitted to the hospital, where he received an intravenous morphine infusion.

Why did he want intravenous medication or even shots when the oral medication was doing its job? Because he is from a culture in which many people believe that the more intrusive the procedure the better it is for them, just as it has been found that many Americans think medicine has to "taste bad" in order for it to be effective.

43   A forty-six-year-old Cambodian woman came into the hospital emergency room complaining of a growth in her abdomen. After five days of testing, the staff finally discovered that Mrs. Sok had not had a bowel movement in ten days. A laxative helped some, but she was not happy with the care she was receiving and did not feel she was getting better. When the physician became aware of her enlarged spleen, he did a bone marrow biopsy. This extremely painful procedure involves inserting a large needle into the bone and aspirating tissue. When the biopsy was completed, Mrs. Sok thanked the doctor profusely, saying she now felt much better.

What accounts for the sudden change in her attitude and perception of her health following this unpleasant procedure? In Cambodia, injections are very common. Since Mrs. Sok had not received one, she felt her care was inadequate and thus she would not get well. She mistook the biopsy for a shot and concluded that she was now on the road to recovery.

There is a lesson from the examples above: It is best to ask the patient what type of medication is preferred, rather than assuming it to be the least invasive form.

Terminology

44   A final note: Be careful about the terminology you use with your patients, even if they are English speaking. Hilda, a nurse working at a cancer center, had a patient with unrelated leg pain. Mrs. Patterson, the patient, was referred to the Pain Team at the center. Hilda was becoming a bit frustrated with Mrs. Patterson because she kept canceling and rescheduling her appointments, while continuing to complain about her pain. When Hilda finally asked her why she wasn't keeping any of her appointments with the Pain Team, Mrs. Patterson replied that she had already suffered enough pain. She didn't need a team to provide her with more!

Once Hilda explained that the Pain Team would only assess her pain and prescribe pain medication, that there was no pain involved in the process, Mrs. Patterson kept her appointment and stopped calling to complain.

Summary

Pain is an unrelenting fact of human life. Although nearly all people experience pain sensations similarly, there are vast cultural differences in the expression of pain. Some cultures encourage the open expression of pain, while others socialize their members to be stoic. Although it is helpful at times to know these generalizations, inaccurate stereotyping can seriously compromise a patient's life. Treat each patient as an individual. The family can also be helpful in letting you know if the patient's behavior is typical or abnormal.

With regard to pain medication, it is often best to anticipate a patient's pain needs, since cultural or religious reasons may inhibit a patient from requesting pain medication even when it is medically necessary for recovery. Also realize that not every patient will share a desire for the least intrusive medication possible. When alternatives are available, it is best to check with the patient; which form would he or she prefer?

For labor pain, see Chapter 9.
For more on medication, see Chapter 12.

Chapter 4
Religion, Beliefs, and Customs

Religion is rarely a topic of conversation in hospitals, but religious beliefs and practices are common sources of conflict and misunderstanding. Patients' exercise of their beliefs can result in amusing or even tragic interference with medical care. This chapter examines both religious and secular beliefs which can create conflicts, misunderstandings—or worse.

Religious Prohibitions

45   A twenty-year-old Buddhist monk from Cambodia was in same day surgery for a hernia repair, accompanied by his mother, aunt, and male cousin. When Lisa, his nurse, entered the room, she greeted him, put her hand on his shoulder, and directed him to a chair across the room. The patient suddenly jumped from her in horror. His mother and aunt lunged at Lisa, shouting at her in Cambodian. Lisa fled the room and called a "code gray," which summoned all male hospital personnel to the area.

When everyone arrived, the cousin was in the corner comforting the patient. Security questioned the patient, but he did not speak enough English to respond. His cousin explained that the patient was a monk and could not be touched by a woman. Should it happen, he was not to look at her, move, or respond in any way. Even a slight tensing of the muscles would be interpreted as showing desire and a breaking of his vows. Because of the incident, he would have to do great penance.

Sadly, this incident could have been avoided. Apparently, the need for strict sexual segregation had been thoroughly discussed with the physician prior to admission. The doctor assured them that there would be no problem. However, he neglected to convey this information to the staff. When questioned, the physician said he thought it would be amusing to see how everyone reacted. It was not. The hospital made arrangements to assure that thereafter the patient would have contact only with males, but the damage had already been done.

The following case study is not one which will be experienced frequently, but it contains many interesting aspects.

His Holiness, the spiritual leader of an Indian Orthodox Christian church, became a patient in an American hospital when he fell ill during a visit to the American Diocese. His condition required cardiac catheterization and open heart surgery. Because it was determined that, despite the extraordinary precautions taken, his body had become contaminated during the procedure, there was a ten-day delay during which he had to undergo a purification ceremony before he could have open heart surgery.

How had he become contaminated? First of all, the surgical team members had allowed non-Orthodox Christians do the electrocardiogram and blood withdrawal and to shave the groin on His Holiness. Priests and bishops within this church must avoid exposing their bodies to any female in order to maintain purity. Although there were no female members directly caring for His Holiness, the director of the catheterization laboratory was a female. Even though she was in the back room, operating the x-ray machines, this was a breach of sexual segregation: His Holiness's private parts had been exposed to a woman.

Although he had not received any food prior to surgery—as is common when anesthesia is used—the medical team allowed him to receive Holy Communion the morning of his heart catheterization. Unfortunately, this led to a cardinal sin. After surgery, His Holiness vomited and the medical team discarded the emesis. Holy Communion is the blood and body of Jesus Christ; when he vomited the Communion, His Holiness was in essence vomiting Christ. The hospital staff should have saved the emesis to be drunk by the priests and bishops there to take care of His Holiness. Drinking the emesis is considered a very holy act, and will wash away one's sins.

The cardiologist in charge of the surgery, himself a member of the church, was held responsible for the breaches of purity. He has been socially isolated from the church as a result. His Holiness's party members, also complicit in the contamination, have probably been banished to remote church monasteries simply because a highly qualified woman was allowed to work the x-ray equipment in the back room and because the hospital staff discarded some vomit.

Although routine sexual segregation is a common practice in many cultures, it is important for health care providers to realize that, in some religious contexts, it is not just a preference but a mandate. If that rule is to be violated in any way—such as allowing a woman to work the x-ray equipment—this should be discussed beforehand. Had the cardi-

46

ologist realized the strength of the church's requirements in the matter, he probably would not have had her at that job. Second, it would be a good idea to go over all possible complications (such as vomiting) to discuss any rules in that regard. Recognizing that rules for religious leaders may be much more stringent than those for others, and ascertaining them in advance, will avoid most of the problems.

Blood Beliefs

Blood Transfusions

47   Susi, a thirty-seven-year-old woman with two children, was horseback riding one day when a snake startled her horse. She was thrown off and landed on a stump, resulting in massive internal injuries. She was rushed to the hospital, where the surgical team discovered that there was a large amount of blood in her abdomen and that she needed to have a kidney removed.

Susi had a medical alert card identifying her as a Jehovah's Witness and stating that under no circumstances was she to receive blood. Her physician knew this, but felt impelled by his oath to save lives to give her a blood transfusion. The hospital was unable to locate Susi's husband, so Dr. Andrews decided to transfuse her.

His actions saved Susi's life; however, Susi was not grateful. She sued her doctor for assault and battery, and won a $20,000 settlement! In a study done of Jehovah's Witnesses in the 1980s, two-thirds of those polled said they would sue if transfused against their will. A physician in a position like that of Dr. Andrews' should realize the possible ramifications (including legal ones) of violating the patients' express wishes in order to fulfill his own beliefs (Hippocratic oath) and make a conscious, fully informed decision.

48   Sometimes a Jehovah's Witness will reconsider at the last minute. For example, a twenty-seven-year-old woman who began bleeding heavily several days after giving birth required a hysterectomy. After the operation, she urgently needed blood but refused it. Two days later, when she developed acute respiratory distress and had to be placed on a respirator, she agreed to the blood transfusion. It saved her life.

Many health care professionals have strong moral difficulty in respecting the Jehovah's Witness position. The conflict lies in two areas: values and world view. The Jehovah's Witnesses believe that when Armageddon comes 144,000 of those who have followed God's laws (as interpreted by the Jehovah's Witnesses) will rise from the dead to spend eternity in heaven. Those who have followed God's laws but do not go to heaven will spend eternity in a paradise on earth. All those who have violated God's laws (e.g., had a blood transfusion, placed themselves above God by celebrating their own birthdays, or worshipped idols by saluting the American flag) are doomed to spend eternity in nothingness.

Suppose for a moment that they are correct. Choosing to have a blood transfusion can be interpreted as giving up the chance to spend eternity in heaven or paradise in exchange for a few more years on earth. In this scenario, it is not very rational to have a blood transfusion. Few health care professionals are Jehovah's Witnesses. They do not believe that the fate of their soul rests on whether they have a blood transfusion. Thus the world view of Jehovah's Witness patients comes into direct conflict with that of most health care professionals.

world view

Most health care professionals value the life of the physical body. In refusing blood, the Jehovah's Witness is valuing the life of the soul over that of the physical body. The question is, Does any group have the right to impose its values and beliefs on others? Can we be so arrogant and ethnocentric as to be sure we are right and they are wrong?

ethos

The issue is most difficult when children are involved. Do their parents have the right to choose for them? This question is not easily answered. In an extreme case, parents abandoned their child after he had been given a blood transfusion under court order.

Finally, there are social issues. If an individual who is a member of a very tightly knit, conservative group of Jehovah's Witnesses accepts blood, the act might lead to rejection by his or her entire social network. A few more years of life may not be worth that price.

social

Why do some members change their mind and accept blood at the last minute? Obviously, not all members of a religion are equally devout. Many people have doubts about their beliefs. When it is a matter of life and death, faith is often not strong enough to dictate the giving up of life.

Dealing with a Jehovah's Witness patient can be very difficult if the need for a blood transfusion arises. Doctors and nurses often feel helpless and frustrated. They value life so strongly that they find it hard to understand why some people willingly choose to give it up. Perhaps they should try to see the situation from the emic perspective and consider the possibility that the Jehovah's Witnesses are right.

Drawing Blood

Saelee Mui Chua, a forty-two-year-old Mien gentleman, arrived at the clinic with his twelve-year-old son, who acted as interpreter. The son explained that his father had seen a traditional healer the previous week, but he had been unable to cure his father's symptoms: weakness, fatigue, increased urination, and thirst. The symptoms suggested dia-

49

betes to the physician, and he ordered a blood glucose test. When Shawnee, the nurse, came to draw the blood, Mr. Saelee fearfully yelled, "No!" His son told Shawnee that his father refused to have his blood drawn. When she asked for an explanation, all he would say is, "My father does not want the test."

The staff assumed that Mr. Saelee was afraid of the needle. However, it is more likely that he was concerned about having his blood drawn. There is a Mien legend about an evil bird that brought bad fortune and death by drinking a person's blood. This is probably connected to the Mien belief that losing blood saps strength (Mr. Saelee was already feeling weak) and may result in the soul leaving the body.

The staff tried to "educate" Mr. Saelee about the procedure of drawing blood, and explained its importance in diagnosing his symptoms, but their efforts were to no avail. He would not give his permission for the procedure and simply left the hospital.

What could have been done? While there are no guarantees that any intervention could have changed Mr. Saelee's mind, they might have explained that the amount of blood needed was extremely small, and that new blood would be made to replace it. If possible, perhaps the traditional healer could have been involved in the procedure. They might have also spent more time explaining why the tests were so necessary. The connection between his symptoms and his blood is not immediately obvious.

Prayer

50   A seventy-five-year-old Black woman named Agnes Jones was in the hospital recovering from a heart attack. Mrs. Jones was very religious and spent most of her time praying. Her "brothers and sisters" from the church visited daily, and she appeared closer to them than to members of her family.

During her hospital stay, Mrs. Jones consented to only the procedures and medications she believed were ordered by God, because according to her world view, only God could make her well. While the nurses bathed Mrs. Jones, she preached to them about Jesus. Before too long, the hospital staff began to avoid her.

For many American Blacks, religion is an essential and integral part of life. God is viewed as the source of both good health and serious illness. God can cure any disease, but to be cured one must pray and have faith. (This world view, like all effective ones, is internally consistent: if a patient is not cured, it is not because God failed but because the patient lacked sufficient faith.)

The hospital personnel did not handle Mrs. Jones's case well. Rather than avoiding her, they should have had a team conference to discuss her beliefs and perhaps invited a minister from her church to attend. The minister might have convinced Mrs. Jones to be more cooperative, and the staff might have learned to be more understanding and tolerant of her beliefs.

In another incident, a Filipino nurse named Erlinda went to check on Inez Said, her Iranian patient. When Erlinda entered the room, she found Mrs. Said huddled on the floor, mumbling. At first she thought Mrs. Said had fallen out of bed, but when she tried to help her up, Mrs. Said became visibly upset. Mrs. Said spoke no English, and Erlinda had no idea what the problem was. At that moment, another nurse walked in. Although she was Anglo, she was married to an East Indian Muslim and was able to explain to Erlinda that Mrs. Said had been praying.

Devout Muslims believe they must pray to Mecca, the Holy Land, five times a day. Traditionally, they pray on a prayer rug placed on the floor. Mrs. Said had been kneeling on such a rug. Though most Muslims in the United States use prayer rugs only in the privacy of their homes, devout Muslims in the Middle East take them when they travel.

Mrs. Said had come to the United States only a week before and was practicing her religion in the traditional manner. Since she was scheduled for surgery the next day, she thought it was especially important to pray.

Throughout the rest of her hospital stay, Mrs. Said refused to acknowledge Erlinda. She evidently felt that Erlinda might have jeopardized the outcome of her surgery by interrupting her prayers. Fortunately, all went well. If the nursing staff had had some understanding of Muslim customs, they could have arranged to give Mrs. Said privacy during certain times of the day so that she could pray.

God or Doctors?

Religious beliefs can interfere with both the acceptance and the administration of particular medical procedures. Emma Chapman, a sixty-two-year-old Black woman, was admitted to the coronary care unit because she had continued episodes of acute chest pain after two heart attacks. Her physician recommended an angiogram with a possible cardiac bypass or angioplasty to follow. Mrs. Chapman refused, saying, "If my faith is strong enough and if it is meant to be, God will cure me."

Although Mrs. Chapman never provided any details, she believed she had sinned and her illness was a punishment. According to her beliefs, illnesses from "natural causes" can be treated through nature (e.g., herbal remedies), but diseases caused by "sin" can be cured only through God's

51

52

intervention. Mrs. Chapman may have felt that to accept medical treatment would be perceived by God as a lack of faith.

Ideally, a staff member would have talked with Mrs. Chapman about her faith, emphasizing that God works through doctors and nurses as well as the patient directly. In this case, medicine could not offer Mrs. Chapman a certain cure; it offered only the possibility of symptom relief and life extension. Someone could have suggested that if she prayed and had enough faith, God would see to it that the operations were successful. She might also have been told the following story:

A huge flood came and destroyed a tiny village. Almost everyone managed to escape in time except for one very religious man who believed that God would save him. He climbed onto his roof to wait. Soon a rescue boat came to help him, but he turned it away, saying, "God will save me." The next day, a second boat came, but again he refused to leave. He said, "My faith in God is strong; He will save me." On the third day, a helicopter flew by to rescue him, and again he turned it away. "God will save me." On the fourth day, the waters rose above his roof and he drowned. When he reached heaven, he demanded to see God. "Why didn't you save me?" he asked. "You've never had a more faithful or loyal servant than I." God responded, "What do you mean? I did try to save you. I sent two boats and a helicopter."

Holy Days

53   Every religion has days that are considered holy and on which behavior is often strictly proscribed. Sol Meyers, an Orthodox Jew, created a problem for the nursing staff when he tried to observe the Sabbath.

Mr. Meyers brought his wife to the hospital in active labor at 8 P.M. on a Friday. When she gave birth at midnight, the nurses suggested that Mr. Meyers accompany her to the postpartum unit and then return home to rest. He thanked them but explained that he could not drive home because it was the Sabbath. The nurses understood and arranged for him to stay in his wife's room.

In the morning, Mr. Meyers asked the nurses for breakfast. They explained that the hospital provided food only for patients; he would have to buy his breakfast in the dining room. When Mr. Meyers told them he was forbidden to ride in an elevator or handle money, one of the nurses offered to get him food. But Mr. Meyers had no money with him. Frustrated, the nurses finally ordered extra food for his wife to share with him. At lunch, Mr. Meyers once again requested food. This time the nurses suggested that he call a friend or relative to pick him up. Mr. Meyers replied that he could not use the phone on the Sabbath, and even if he made a call, no one would answer because all his friends and relatives were Orthodox. By this time, the nurses were losing patience. If Mr. Meyers could drive to the hospital, why couldn't he drive home? If he knew he would have to stay at the hospital, why had he not brought food with him?

The answers can be found in the Torah. One of the most important laws of the Torah states that Orthodox Jews must observe the Sabbath. It is a time to be with one's family and to worship God. The Sabbath begins at sundown Friday and ends at sundown Saturday. During this time, work of any kind is prohibited, including driving, using the telephone, handling money, and even pushing an elevator button. (A large Jewish hospital in Los Angeles features a few elevators that automatically stop on every floor on Saturday.)

The only law higher than the law of the Sabbath is the law that demands one do everything possible to save a life. Mr. Meyers could drive his wife to the hospital on the Sabbath because her life and that of their child were at stake. He could not drive home, however, because a life was not threatened. Mr. Meyers did not bring food with him because it is forbidden to travel with food on the Sabbath (unless it is milk for a baby). Very little else could have been done in this situation other than to charge extra food to the patient's bill.

In another situation involving Jews, a young boy was severely injured one Saturday afternoon while playing football. He needed to go to the hospital immediately. The only person available to take him was his Orthodox grandfather, who drove him the twenty-five miles to the hospital. Once the boy was safely admitted, his grandfather walked home.

54

Sacred Symbols

Religious and spiritual symbols are not always obvious to members of other religions, and this can lead to problems. In one case, an emergency room patient named Maria Burlatti needed a chest x-ray. When the technician removed her gown, he found a rosary around Mrs. Burlatti's neck and asked her to remove it. Mrs. Burlatti was Italian and spoke very little English. Realizing that she did not understand his request, the technician attempted to remove the rosary himself, whereupon Mrs. Burlatti became extremely upset and slapped him. A nursing student tried to explain to the patient through gestures that her rosary would be returned as soon as the x-rays were completed, but she still did not understand. She began to cry.

55

The head nurse then came upon the scene. She sat beside Mrs. Burlatti and quietly explained why the rosary had to be removed. Although she understood the words no better than those of the technician and student nurse, Mrs. Burlatti responded to the calm and soothing voice.

The head nurse gently lifted the rosary off her neck and placed it on top of Mrs. Burlatti's head. The rosary thus remained in contact with her body but did not get in the way of the x-rays.

The technician, who was not Catholic, did not realize the rosary was a religious item and assumed it was a necklace. The patient, who was ill and scared, needed the symbol of her religious faith more than ever. Although most Catholics do not wear rosaries, hospital personnel should realize that older Italian and Mexican women may.

56 Abby, a nurse who worked at a hospital close to the Hoopa Indian reservation in Northern California, told of an elderly Native American man in intensive care. His granddaughter brought in an object consisting of a circular frame with feathers hanging from it. The object fits the description of a "soul catcher." She asked if she could hang it on the wall. Fortunately, Abby was quite understanding and took it and hung it from the intravenous hook above the patient's bed instead. The granddaughter was both relieved and grateful. It was a small concession on the part of the nurse, but provided tremendous psychological comfort for the patient and his family.

57 A Cambodian infant was brought into the hospital diagnosed with dehydration 5 percent. Mona, the nurse, examined the child's extremities, looking for a vein in which to start an intravenous line. She found one on the baby's arm. At that point, she noticed several strands of dark brown strings, about one-half inch wide, on both wrists. Mona prepared to cut the strings with scissors. Mrs. Tep, the baby's mother, walked in at that moment, looked horrified at what Mona was about to do, and began speaking loudly in her native tongue. Mona assumed she was upset because the infant was crying. But Mrs. Tep kept pointing to the strings; it was obvious that she did not want them cut. Mona did not understand what the problem was, but communicated through gestures that she would not cut the strings.

She then started an intravenous line in the infant's scalp. When the baby's parents saw this, the mother began to cry. While it is distressing for any parent to see intravenous lines put into a sick child's scalp, for many Southeast Asians, it is especially traumatic. As the Teps explained through an interpreter, the head is thought to be the seat of life. By introducing holes into it, the nurse had made an easy exit for the child's soul.

What was the problem with the strings? They are known as *baci*. It is a tradition believed to have originated with the Lao culture, but is practiced by the Mien and Cambodians as well. The strings are tied around a person's wrists at important occasions—birthdays, promotions, weddings, and so forth. They are believed to "tie in the soul" so it doesn't get lost. They should never be cut off; they simply wear off in time. If Mona had cut the strings, she would have jeopardized the infant's life from the Tepses' perspective.

A general rule of thumb is to assume that a patient who is wearing anything that looks unusual may be doing so for religious or spiritual reasons. Hindus may wear sacred threads around their necks or arms; Native Americans may carry medicine bundles; Mexican children may wear a bit of red ribbon; Mediterranean peoples may wear a special charm on a chain, such as a mustard seed in a blue circle or a ram's horn, to ward off the evil eye. If an item must be removed to perform a medical procedure, the reason should be explained to the patient and the family. The item should be removed gently and respectfully and kept in contact with the patient's body if possible.

The Garment

Grace Kettering, a Mormon woman, was admitted to the hospital for facial surgery. Before entering the operating room, she was told to re- move all her clothes except the hospital gown. She refused to remove her long underwear, and the surgeon refused to operate unless she did.   58

Devout Mormons who have attained adult religious status in the church wear "the garment." It resembles short-sleeved long underwear and ends just above the knee. Although not exactly magical, it is con- sidered sacred and is always worn except when being cleaned or while one is bathing. Having to remove the garment associated with God's protection can be very distressing to a Mormon patient, especially prior to surgery.

Eventually, Mrs. Kettering's surgeon relented. In such cases, an un- derstanding attitude and a discussion of the options beforehand are advisable. For example, the lower half of the garment could be pulled down to the patient's ankles in the event of abdominal surgery.

Evil Eye

Belief in the evil eye is widespread throughout Central America, the Mediterranean, the Middle East, much of Africa, and parts of Asia. Al- though the beliefs and associated practices vary, the concept generally includes an evil that one puts on another that causes the victim to fall ill. The motive is usually envy.

Anthropologists have explained the evil eye curse in terms of the "theory of limited good," which is based on the idea that there is a lim- ited amount of good things in the world, whether beauty, intelligence, wealth, luck, or health. If one person gets more, there is less of it in the world for others. Envy may dictate giving someone the evil eye. The victim's ensuing illness somehow helps even things out.

Belief in the evil eye can create distress and confusion between Mexican and American mothers. In Mexican culture, babies are considered weak and extremely susceptible to the power of an envious glance. It is not even necessary to wish a child harm; a simple compliment, unaccompanied by a touch, can bring on the evil eye. Touching the person while complimenting him or her, however, neutralizes the power of the evil eye.

59   Sue Ramis, a home health nurse, received an angry call from Juanita Garcia, a Mexican American woman whose house she had visited the day before. As Sue was leaving, she innocently remarked that Mrs. Garcia's child was adorable. The next morning, the infant was crying and feverish. When Mrs. Garcia recalled Sue's compliment and the fact that she had not touched the child, she concluded that Sue had given him the evil eye. Being Anglo, Sue had no knowledge of evil eye. She was innocent, except in the mind of Mrs. Garcia.

Americans are raised to believe that germs cause disease. Mothers are uncomfortable when people get too close to their infants. Mexican mothers, in contrast, may worry when strangers admire their babies without touching them. The very act that is believed to protect a child from illness in one culture is thought to cause illness in another.

Each culture that believes compliments can cause the evil eye also has ways to neutralize them. Putting a bit of saliva on one's finger and making the sign of the cross on a child's forehead when giving a compliment can prevent the evil eye in some (but not all) parts of the Philippines. In Ethiopia, spitting on a child while remarking on its good looks will prevent an inadvertent casting of the evil eye. Not all Mexicans, Filipinos, or Ethiopians adhere to the belief, however, so it is important to pay close attention to nonverbal cues from the mother. Does she appear uncomfortable when you compliment her child? If so, she may believe in the evil eye.

Soul Loss

60   Melissa was working in a busy pediatric intensive care unit the day she inadvertently jeapordized Jimmy Hosea's life. Jimmy was a twelve-year-old post-op Navaho patient. The day he transferred into Melissa's unit, the staff had just been given a new Polaroid camera. She gathered together Jimmy and two other children for a photo. Because her attention was on the two others who happily mugged for the camera, Melissa

never noticed the look of horror on Jimmy's face until she saw the photo. He had disappeared while it was developing.

When Melissa found him, Jimmy was sitting on the edge of his bed, gazing at the floor and looking as though he were ready to die. When she asked him what had happened, he carefully responded, "I've lost my soul." Melissa had no idea what he was talking about. He explained that pictures took the soul out of the face captured on the photograph. Melissa was astounded. How could he believe that?

She told him how sorry she was and offered him the photograph. He took it, saying that his family could help him get his soul back with a "sing," a religious ceremony.

This case is a good example of how important it is to know about the spiritual beliefs of those for whom you are caring. While it is obviously unrealistic to expect to know everything about every culture, just having an awareness that your patients' beliefs may be different from your own may help you to be more sensitive and aware. Melissa certainly is.

Lucky and Unlucky Numbers

In Chinese and Japanese languages, the character for the number "4" is pronounced the same as the word for "death," and thus may create some discomfort for Chinese and Japanese patients. This number will be discussed in more detail in Chapter 10. Other numbers have significance as well. Recall that many Americans are superstitious about the number 13. In fact, many buildings lack a thirteenth floor, and many hospitals go from room 12 to room 14 on all wards. Different numbers have positive or negative associations in other cultures.

The Chinese regard numbers 8 and 9 as lucky. The character for 8 signifies wealth and the character for 9 means long life. In Hong Kong, most of the expensive luxury cars owned by the Chinese include the number 8 on the license plate. The Chinese pay extra money and wait in long lines to get a plate with that number. An expensive car without an 8 is generally owned by a foreigner.

Whereas the number 4 has negative connotations for the Japanese, the opposite is the case for the Navaho, who see much of the world in terms of four. Phrases are repeated four times in their ritual chants, pollen is thrown to the four directions in many of their ceremonies, and they revere four sacred mountains. A Navaho might find it easier to remember to take medicine four times a day than three or five times.

Obviously, health care workers cannot be expected to know all the superstitions of every ethnic group. What is important to remember is that superstitions are a part of every culture and may surface during the emotionally trying times of illness. Problems can be avoided by giving patients as much information as possible in advance and then by being sensitive to their reactions.

The Right Hand

61   Issam Khattab was an Arab student at an American university. He had a perforated colon and needed a temporary colostomy. Sylvia was the nurse assigned to teach him how to use the pouch applied over the surgical opening on his bowel. Sylvia was surprised to find Issam noncompliant when it came to learning how to perform his self-care with the pouch. The main problem is that he would only use one hand to open and rinse out the pouch; he refused to use both hands. Since it was extremely difficult to do one-handed, he would always call Sylvia to empty the pouch. Sylvia warned him of the dangers of having the unemptied pouch burst, but he still refused to empty it. Finally, to "teach him a lesson," she let it burst. Issam, now covered with his own feces, was angry and embarrassed, but at last began to care for himself.

Why was he so stubborn? Probably because in the Arab tradition, one uses one's right hand to eat and one's left hand to clean after going to the bathroom. Since food in much of the Middle East is traditionally eaten with one's hand out of a communal bowl, it is an important hygiene measure that people use separate hands for separate tasks. Most likely, Issam was avoiding using his right hand to clean his pouch. It is unfortunate that he did not explain the situation to Sylvia; she could have used disposable pouches which he could change using only one hand. Since that incident, she has done just that with her patients who are reluctant to perform the necessary maintenance of their pouches.

Hair

62   Raj Singh, a seventy-two-year-old Sikh from India, had been admitted to the hospital after a heart attack. He was scheduled for a heart catheterization to determine the extent of the blockage in his coronary arteries. The procedure involved running a catheter up the femoral artery, located in the groin, and then passing it into his heart where special x-rays could be taken. His son was a cardiologist on staff and had explained the procedure to him in detail.

Susan, his nurse, entered Mr. Singh's room and explained that she had to shave his groin to prevent infection from the catheterization. As she pulled the razor from her pocket, she was suddenly confronted with the sight of shining metal flashing in front of her. Mr. Singh had a short sword in his hand and was waving it at her as he spoke excitedly in his native tongue. Susan got the message. She would not shave his groin.

She put away her "weapon," and he did the same. Susan, thinking the problem was that she was a woman, said she would get a male orderly to shave him. Mr. Singh's eyes lit up again as he angrily yelled, "No shaving of hair by anyone!"

Susan managed to calm him down by agreeing. She then called her supervisor and the attending physician to report the incident. The physician said he would do the procedure on an unshaved groin. At that moment, Mr. Singh's son stopped by. When he heard what had happened, he apologized profusely for not explaining his father's Orthodox Sikh customs.

The Sikh religion forbids cutting or shaving any bodily hair. Orthodox Sikhs always carry a dagger with them, lest someone try to force them to do something against their religion—as Susan had. The dagger is considered one of the five "outer badges." The others are wearing hair and beard unshorn; wearing a turban; wearing knee-length pants; and wearing a steel bracelet on the right wrist. These badges reflect the Sikhs' military history.

Many of the procedures medical professionals consider necessary are not; when they conflict with patients' religious beliefs, they can be worked around. The doctor might have been willing to make compromises in Mr. Singh's case only because his son was a member of the staff. All patients should be treated with the same respect.

A Native American woman named Estelle Begay brought her fifteen-month-old granddaughter Elena into the emergency room. The child was suffering from severe dehydration and fever. To restore fluids intravenously, the nurse shaved Elena's right temple and inserted an intravenous line. Mrs. Begay was busy completing admitting papers while this was done. When she reached the unit to see her granddaughter, she became very anxious and upset. The nurse tried to reassure her that the intravenous lines were temporary and that as soon as the problem was corrected, the child would be fine. Mrs. Begay responded with sorrow and resignation. "She's going to die." The nurse tried to reassure her, but Mrs. Begay would not leave Elena's bedside.

At one point, Mrs. Begay did leave for a few hours. She returned with two relatives and a "medicine bundle," which she tried to put on Elena's bed. This was against hospital policy, however, and was not permitted. The nurse said she could leave it by the window, if she desired.

Mrs. Begay and the other relatives, who were no longer permitted in the unit except during limited visiting hours, kept a vigil outside the door. The next day, despite Elena's improvement, Mrs. Begay insisted on taking her home against medical advice.

63

The following day, Elena was readmitted by her mother. She was still feverish and would not eat. A small bundle was attached to the child's shirt. As the nurse started to remove it, the mother stopped her. "Please let her keep it. It is our custom." She went on to explain why Mrs. Begay had taken the child home against medical advice. She was afraid Elena would die.

"In our culture, it is taboo to cut a child's hair. Long, thick hair is a sign of a healthy child. To cut or shave it means the child will become sick or die." Mrs. Begay had obtained a medicine bundle to counteract the effect of violating the taboo but was not permitted to put it next to the child. It was useless sitting by the window. Mrs. Begay had no recourse but to take Elena home, where she could use the curative charm. This time, the nurses agreed to let the medicine bundle be placed next to Elena. After four days, her condition improved and she was able to go home.

This example illustrates two important points. The first is the same discussed above under religious and spiritual symbols—do not remove them. Second, many cultures have prohibitions against cutting hair, as was illustrated in the case involving Mr. Singh. The biblical tale of Samson, who lost his strength when his hair was cut, reflects a similar taboo.

Bathing

64   Niki's eyes rolled when she saw her patient, Mr. Johnson. "Another street person," she thought. It wasn't that she had anything against the homeless, the problem was that they just didn't like to bathe. As a nurse, she thought cleanliness was next to godliness. Sure enough, when she tried to bathe Mr. Johnson, he became visibly upset. "No, no." When she asked him why, he explained that the layer of dirt would help to protect him from illness.

Although this belief is in direct contraction with Western medicine, it is easy to see why it would be adaptive for people living on the street to develop a belief which is consistent with their circumstances, specifically, greatly reduced access to bathing facilities.

Niki wished she could just force him to bathe, but she knew she couldn't; it was a matter of patients' rights. Only if he had to have surgery could she make him take a shower. She sighed and reminded herself that it was a question of beliefs and values, and she shouldn't impose hers on others.

Summary

Although conflicting belief systems can be a source of frustration, confusion, and misunderstanding, most can be dealt with successfully. One must understand the patient's beliefs and be willing to respect them. When health care personnel work *with* the patient's beliefs, rather than against them, the outcomes are usually more successful, measured not only in patient satisfaction but also in ease for the medical team in managing the patient and family.

Chapter 5
Dietary Practices

Dietary practices are an important concern for hospitals. Patients are often misdiagnosed as lacking in appetite because they refuse hospital foods. Families frequently bring in traditional foods for patients, which may in fact be harmful to their condition. Knowledge of cultural differences in dietary rules and food preferences is essential both in terms of patient satisfaction and health.

Ramadan

65 Ali, the thirty-year-old son of a Saudi oil prince, refused to eat the food on his meal tray. Throughout the night, however, he would request that the nurses bring him fruits and vegetables. The staff was becoming annoyed with his odd eating patterns, until they learned that is was the month of Ramadan, an important Muslim religious festival. During that time followers are forbidden to eat from sunrise to sunset. Although for many Muslims illness provides an exemption from the rules, try to accommodate devout Muslim patients as much as possible without compromising their health.

Kosher Dietary Practices

66 Why would a fifty-four-year-old man burst into tears when served meat, milk, and butter on the same lunch tray? What would cause an eighty-seven-year-old woman to refuse beef and chicken, even though she was not a vegetarian? Why would the mother of a two-year-old patient refuse to use the flatware provided and instead insist on plastic utensils? All these individuals are Orthodox Jews following the kosher dietary laws. These laws forbid eating pork and shellfish and nonkosher red meat and poultry, and mixing meat and dairy products, either in the same meal or by using the same plates, pots, or utensils for both.

As with most cultural and religious laws, there is a practical and ideological basis for their origin. The overriding ideology behind the kosher laws is humaneness. The practical reasons are generally associated with health.

Shellfish are to be avoided because they are scavengers. They can pick up cause trichinosis. Furthermore, pigs require shade, water, and human food. In the desert environment it is not a good idea to raise animals that compete with humans for scarce resources. The last two points might explain why Muslims also forbid eating pork. An alternative explanation suggests that because pork and shellfish were dietary staples in the lands where the Jews lived at different points in their history, the taboo was designed to prevent the Jews from integrating. For meat to be considered kosher, animals must be killed with a single blow and not strangled. The pain and suffering an animal experiences between the first and final blows or during the time it takes to die from strangulation can stimulate the release of hormones detrimental to humans. Finally, a common supposition is that if meat and dairy products are combined, bits of meat may lodge in a wooden or pottery bowl, mix with the dairy products, and in the desert sun provide an ideal breeding ground for bacteria.

Again, the notion of humaneness underlies most of the kosher laws. One can get milk from a living cow or goat, eggs from a living chicken, and wool from a living sheep, but pigs are useful only when dead. To raise an animal strictly for slaughter is considered cruel and inhumane, as is mixing the meat of a calf with the milk of its mother. Finally, the most humane death is one that is instantaneous.

The practical reasons for most of the kosher laws no longer exist. Yet Orthodox Jews continue to uphold the traditions. The behavior of the patients described earlier becomes clear in light of these laws. All these situations can be easily avoided through knowledge of these kosher laws and the use of readily available frozen kosher meal trays and nonreusable paper plates and plastic utensils.

Beef

Christy, an Anglo nurse, took pity on the elderly man in the emergency room. He had been there for hours and appeared hungry. She went out of her way to get him a hamburger. When she gave it to him, his son, rather than appear grateful, was angry. His father was Hindu, and therefore forbidden to eat beef. She would have been wise to offer him a few alternatives prior to getting him food.

Dietary Practices: Hot and Cold

68   Nonreligious food restrictions can also create problems. Mina Asami, a sixty-seven-year-old Pakistani woman, was hospitalized with tuberculosis. When Rachel, her nurse, noticed that Mrs. Asami's appetite was poor, she became concerned. Wanting to make sure her patient received enough protein, she made a concerted effort to feed her meat and potatoes with gravy. Mrs. Asami, however, was uncooperative, eating only fruit and Jello.

When Mrs. Asami's son Davi came to the hospital, he provided information that resolved the problem. Rachel, it appears, was trying to feed Mrs. Asami foods that Pakistanis normally avoid during the summer. Foods are either hot or cold. These are qualities, not temperatures. In the summer, Pakistanis avoid hot foods like beef because they "make our insides hot." In winter, they avoid cold foods that make their insides cold. Beef, pork, potatoes, and whiskey are all considered hot foods and are avoided in summer; in winter, Pakistanis refrain from eating cold foods such as chicken, fish, fruit, and beer. Once Rachel understood this, she ordered the appropriate foods for Mrs. Asami, who suddenly developed a much heartier appetite.

69   It is best to ask about food preferences during the admission interview or to arrange for a family member to bring food in for the patient. The latter approach was taken by the family of Chi-Wa Koo, a Chinese patient with lung cancer. A complete Chinese kitchen was laid out on a hospital serving cart. Mr. Koo refused to eat anything prepared by the hospital, consuming only those items brought and prepared by his family.

Mr. Koo's family regarded his lung cancer as a *yin* or cold condition. To restore balance to his system, it was necessary to give him *yang* or hot foods. Without a knowledge of *yin* and *yang*, it would be impossible for the hospital to serve Mr. Koo the appropriate foods. Furthermore, in China, the family traditionally supplies a patient's food. Fortunately, this incident occurred in a national medical center that is used to treating patients from all over the world. The staff willingly accommodated Mr. Koo's needs by allowing his family to bring in his food.

Food Preferences

Each ethnic group has its own food preferences. Filipinos, for example, like rice with every meal and may feel deprived without it. They sometimes say it is a great comfort to eat rice when they feel ill. Food preferences should be ascertained when a patient is admitted and checked throughout hospitalization because they can have an important psychological effect. Simply discussing the daily menu with the patient can make a significant difference in the patient's attitude and recovery.

Mrs. Vu, a Vietnamese refugee in her late sixties, was brought to the   70
hospital by her sponsor for observation. She was tired and losing weight.
Her tests were all negative, however. The nurses tried to get Mrs. Vu to
eat, but without success. Fortunately, a Vietnamese dietitian had recently
been hired. When consulted, she asked the nurses what kind of food they
had offered Mrs. Vu. She had been given beefsteak, mashed potatoes,
vegetables, cherry cobbler, milk, and coffee, then considered to be a
healthy, well-balanced meal—for an American, that is. Mrs. Vu had
never eaten foods prepared in this way. When they gave her rice and
vegetables stir-fried with beef, she ate everything on her plate, a simple
solution to her dietary problem.

Mrs. Nyguen, the sixty-five-year-old Vietnamese refugee described in   71
Chapter 2, was dehydrated and malnourished. She was receiving pallia-
tive care for cancer. She ate little and did not comply with the dietitian's
recommended liquid supplement.

While interviewing the patient regarding her condition and health
care practices, Martha, the home health nurse, learned that she was not
taking the dietary supplement that the dietitian had recommended. Martha realized that it was in the form of a sweet-tasting shake, agreeable to
the Western palate but not to her client. She spoke with the dietitian and
obtained a non-sweet substitute, which the client found much more to
her liking. She said the taste was similar to that of rice-water.

It is important to realize that people of different cultures prefer different "tastes"; noncompliance may simply be a result of unpalatable
flavors.

Dietary Problems

Some ethnic groups cannot tolerate certain foods. According to some
studies, most Asians, Blacks, and Native Americans are lactose intolerant,
and milk products give them gas and diarrhea. Calcium needs should be
considered, however, in planning meals for pregnant women, whether
in the hospital or at home. Calcium supplements may be necessary.
Other foods such as tofu, collard greens, bok choy, and sardines, all of
which are high in calcium, should be emphasized. Hispanics generally
consider pregnancy a hot condition. Protein-rich foods, which are also
usually hot, are avoided during pregnancy to maintain body balance.
Physicians should take special care to make sure such women receive
adequate protein.

Typical ethnic diets must also be taken into account when discharging
patients with special dietary requirements. Asian diets are generally very
low in fats but high in sodium. Mexican Americans tend to use a lot of
salt and fats in their cooking. Either of these ethnic cooking styles could

prove problematic for hypertensive patients. It may be unrealistic to expect someone to change cooking and eating styles completely. Teaching sessions or adjustment of medications may be necessary. The family cook should be included in all discussions.

Food Deprivation

72   An Anglo nurse working in Saudi Arabia encountered a potentially life-threatening dietary problem involving many of her hemodialysis patients. Dates, a favorite food of many Arabs, are very high in potassium, which must be strictly limited in someone suffering from kidney failure. The nurse could not always find an interpreter to explain the situation clearly and convincingly to patients. The situation was further complicated, first, because in Saudi Arabia, food deprivation is considered a precursor to illness. From an Arab perspective, the nurses were helping to bring on illness by depriving patients of dates. Second, Muslims believe that Allah (God) is all-powerful. Neither dates nor potassium would influence their health; rather, it was God's will. *Inshallah.* If Allah meant them to die, so be it. If not, they would survive. Beyond patient teaching, there is little one can do in such a situation.

Summary

Food is essential to health, yet the traditional diets of many patients may conflict with standard hospital fare. As a result, patients may refuse to eat, which can both compromise their health and confuse their diagnosis. It is advisable for health care personnel to have some knowledge of traditional diets, both in terms of content and preparation, and to involve the patient or family in designing meals. In an era of increasing competition between hospitals for patients, it is the savvy hospital that will make accommodations to the patients' preferred diet.

Chapter 6
Family

When asked to name their most common problem in dealing with non-Anglo ethnic groups, most nurses respond, "their families."

Visitors

A sixty-five-year-old Filipino woman named Carlita Ricos lay dying for six months. Although she was in a coma, her fourteen children were with her constantly, bathing her, grooming her, rubbing her favorite lotion on her skin. Her failure to respond did nothing to diminish their devotion. The nursing staff reacted in several ways. Many were impressed with the dedication of the Ricos family. Others were annoyed by the constant stream of visitors. Few understood why Mrs. Ricos's family spent so much time with her.

Filipinos have great respect for their parents. They feel they owe an eternal debt of prime obligation—*utang na loob*—to their parents for giving them life and making sacrifices for them. Mrs. Ricos's children felt they owed their mother all the time and care they could give. They never considered that they might be in the nurses' way.

A similar incident involved a Chinese family. Very early one morning, before the sun had arisen, Chi-Fan Wong's nurse, Nancy, stumbled over a body curled up on the floor. When her eyes grew accustomed to the darkness, she discovered two other people sleeping on a cot and in the chair. Mr. Wong's wife was standing at his bedside, holding her husband's glass while he swallowed his medications. Nancy soon discovered a serving cart filled with food prepared by his family. Later that afternoon, another group of family members arrived and the original group went home to rest.

Until the night Mr. Wong died, someone was with him at all times. The visitor's chair served as a bed. His wife and sons bathed him, fed him, and massaged his body. Interestingly, his sons were more involved in his

75   care than his daughters. In an almost identical situation, Sam Inouye, a Japanese patient in his late fifties, was constantly attended by his wife and children. They took over all his personal care, a service usually provided by the nurses.

The custom in both China and Japan is for the family to take care of the patient's personal needs. The medical staff is there to practice medicine. Both respect and obligation require that children minister to their parents.

The Asian respect for parents can be illustrated by the following hypothetical situation. You are in a boat with your mother and your child when the boat capsizes. You can save only one person. Whom do you save? Most Americans would respond, "My child," reasoning that their mother had lived her life whereas their child's was just beginning. Most Asians perceive the situation differently. They would more likely respond, "My mother," explaining that they can always have another child, but they can have only one mother. (Nigerians ask a similar question, but the boat's occupants are your mother and your *wife*. The culturally "correct" response is the same as that described for Asians!)

The different perspectives also reflect a difference in family relationships. Traditionally, most Asians live in extended family households and tend to value the family of orientation (the individual, parents, and siblings) above the family of procreation (the individual, spouse, and children). Sons generally live with their parents until they die, and that long-term relationship takes precedence over any other. In contrast, Americans usually live in nuclear family households. Ties to parents are weakened after marriage, while those to spouse and children are strengthened. The choice whether to save the mother or child reflects the traditionally stronger familial tie.

The reason Mr. Wong's sons were more involved in his care than his daughters is that Chinese were traditionally patrilocal; that is, sons continued to live with their parents after marriage. It was their obligation to care for their aging progenitors. Daughters, however, moved in with their in-laws. Their primary responsibility was to their husbands' parents, not their own. Therefore, in an extension of traditional residence patterns, we find the man's sons at his bedside, rather than his daughters.

76   Asians are not the only ethnic group that hovers around the sick beds of their relatives. The entire family of a sixteen-year-old Mexican American youth crowded in the hospital waiting room while he was being treated for minor injuries. A friend had brought him into the emergency room at 1:30 A.M. He had been injured in a gang fight. Fortunately, the contusions and lacerations he received were not serious; few stitches were required. Nevertheless, well over a dozen relatives—including aunts,

uncles, and cousins—arrived at the hospital and remained by his side until he was released.

Gypsies cause some of the worst complaints regarding family visitors. For example, when Louis Romano, king of his clan, became ill, thirty to fifty of his relatives, friends, and "elders" literally took over the small hospital where he was a patient in intensive care. They came in the evening and stayed all night, despite the posted notice that visiting hours were limited. The Gypsies who were not in the patient's room or lobby roamed the parking lot. Everyone in the hospital—supervisors, security, maintenance, office staff, and nurses—tried in vain to maintain order, politely explaining procedure and protocol, but without effect.   77

Gypsies live within a large extended family unit known as a clan. All members are considered immediate family. When any member is ill, it is important to show respect and concern through one's presence. Because the patient in this case was the king, the attendance of the entire clan was almost mandatory. A few elders even came from across the country to be with him.

Gypsies are commonly nomadic, traveling in groups. When they enter a hospital, that becomes their temporary home. If possible, Gypsy patients should be put in private rooms at the end of a hall so as to minimize traffic problems and disturbance to other patients. Other than that, hospital staff must be prepared for a constant stream of people moving into the hospital to be near the patient.

One reason large numbers of ethnic family members who visit patients and often remain twenty-four hours a day create significant difficulties for hospital staff is that American hospitals were built by Americans for Americans. Americans tend to have small families and to live in nuclear family households. Furthermore, privacy is a major American value. Generally few family members live near enough to the hospital to come visit very often. When they do, they usually stay for only a short period of time because they feel the patient should be left alone to rest in order to get well. Therefore, hospital rooms rarely have more than one visitor's chair per bed and visiting hours may be extremely limited. Second, Americans value money as well as privacy. Hospitals are a business. If there is room for another bed, it should be for a patient, not for a family member who wants to sleep over.

Hospitals in other cultures are designed and run differently. Patients are expected to have several visitors. A cot is usually provided for anyone who spends the night. Privacy is not a concern.

Betsy Sanders, a former student, broke her leg in a skiing accident in Spain. The doctor at the clinic told Betsy that her ligaments were shredded but that he could correct the condition with surgery. When Betsy   78 awoke from surgery, she was nauseated and in terrible pain but could not vomit. She was too embarrassed. There were ten people in the room waiting to see her. She was in a large private room, and a couch had been turned into a guest bed. All her friends in Spain had gotten together and decided Betsy should never be left alone. They worked out a visiting schedule. One friend even took a leave of absence from work to be with her.

Although Betsy appreciated their concern, their solicitousness made her uncomfortable. All but one of her friends were male. She was in bed with her leg in the air for two weeks, wearing nothing but a little gown. She had to be washed in bed and use a bedpan. She could not wash her hair or even brush her teeth. She looked awful and felt worse. All she wanted was to be left alone.

Her situation was the reverse of the non-Anglo in an American hospital. The hospital staff expected her to have visitors around the clock and provided a bed for that purpose. Her friends assumed she would want company and ignored what they interpreted as her polite protestations that she would be fine if left alone. She did not have any family in Spain so they were filling in. They would have wanted the same attention had the situation been reversed. In this case, however, what the patient longed for was some privacy.

79   A young Lebanese nurse changed her attitude toward family visitors when she herself became a patient. The evening she had surgery, eight relatives came in a group to see her. It made her feel good to be the object of so much love and support. At the same time, she realized that had she been the nurse in this case, she would have felt that the large number of visitors was unacceptable, and would have asked them to leave. She had done this before with other patients, thinking that it was for the patient's own good. She realized that, in the past, she might have mistakenly imposed the values of the health care system on her patients.

What she learned from this experience was to talk to her patients about their feelings regarding visitors before the visitors arrived. Then she could truly do what was best for her patient.

In summary, then, hospitals are designed with the needs and values of the culture in mind. Problems arise when the patient is of a different ethnic group, with a different set of values and needs. In a country like the United States, with its huge population of non-Anglo residents, this is frequently the case. It is important to remember that the patient is not just an individual but a member of a family. When one member is ill, the entire group is affected. Ideally, the family can help care for the patient, freeing the staff for more technical medical care.

A related problem that frequently arises is the failure of many non-Anglo patients to care for themselves.

Self-Care

Tome Tanaka, a Japanese man in his sixties, was a patient in the reha-   80
bilitation unit. A stroke had left him with significant weakness on his left
side. Self-care was an important part of his therapy. He had to relearn
to feed himself, dress, shave, use the bathroom, and do other daily activities. Kathy, his nurse, spent a great deal of time carefully explaining
to Mr. Tanaka how the staff would work with him on these tasks. The
patient and his wife listened passively; his children and grandchildren
appeared more interested. Several hours later, when Mr. Tanaka's children and grandchildren left, Kathy came into the room and discovered
Mrs. Tanaka waiting on her husband as though he were an invalid.

She was not alone in impeding his progress, however. He refused
to do anything for himself and continually barked commands at her.
Rather than use the toilet, he insisted that she hold the bedpan for him.
He refused to brush his teeth, shave, or dress, demanding that his wife
do everything for him.

Mr. Tanaka attended physical therapy and occupational therapy sessions each day and did quite well. He learned to walk with a cane. He
needed minimal assistance with self-care activities. Despite his progress
in therapy, however, as soon as his wife or one of his children arrived, he
regressed. He was discharged after four weeks, almost as dependent as
when he first came.

Kathy and the other nurses were frustrated over Mr. Tanaka's depen-
dency, especially when they saw that he was capable of taking care of
himself. They took his "failure" personally, as though they were not doing their jobs properly. What might the nurses have done differently?
First, they needed to understand that patients and their families do
not always share the same goals as health care personnel. Second, they
might have allowed the family to observe Mr. Tanaka during physical and
occupational therapy sessions. Unlike most hospitals, this one barred
families from such sessions because of the potential distraction for the
patient. In this case, the rule might have been waived.

Juan Martinez, a thirty-six-year-old Mexican man with second degree   81
burns on his hands and arms, posed a similar problem. The skin grafts
had healed, and there was now danger that the area would stiffen
and the tissue shorten. The only way to maintain maximum mobility
was through regular stretching and exercise. The nurses explained to
Mr. Martinez's wife that feeding himself was an essential therapeutic exercise. The act of grasping the utensils and lifting the food to the mouth
stretches the necessary areas. Mrs. Martinez seemed to understand the
nurses' explanation, yet she continued to cut her husband's food and put
it in his mouth.

When Linda, one of his nurses, observed this, she took the fork out of Mrs. Martinez's hand and told Mr. Martinez to feed himself because he needed to exercise his arms and hands. Linda again explained to Mr. Martinez's wife how important it was for him to do it himself. Mrs. Martinez appeared skeptical but did not argue. Mr. Martinez looked at Linda peevishly and made a feeble attempt at eating. His wife watched with pity. Linda knew from seeing Mr. Martinez when his wife was not around that he was perfectly capable of feeding himself. Linda left the room. When she looked in five minutes later, she saw Mrs. Martinez once again cutting her husband's food and putting it in his mouth.

Failure to care for oneself is common in cultures that emphasize the family over the individual—in other words, almost all cultures other than Anglo-American. Self-care is important to Americans in part because we value independence so highly. In contrast, Asian and Hispanic cultures emphasize family interdependence over independence. For them, self-care is not an important concept.

In many cases, Americans' ethnocentrism blinds them to the fact that life in a typical Asian or Hispanic household may be different from that in the normal Anglo home. Self-care may be a practical necessity in the Anglo home, where there may be no one to help the former patient with such tasks. In contrast, many Asians and Hispanics live in large extended family households, where someone is usually at home to care for the patient.

Another significant factor is the difference between egalitarian and hierarchical cultures. In an egalitarian culture such as our own, everyone is theoretically equal. And, theoretically, no one in the family is considered subservient to anyone else. In hierarchical Asian cultures, some members of the family are clearly dominant (males and elders) while others are clearly subordinate (females and children). The case study involving the Tanakas illustrates the proper roles of wife and children in hierarchical cultures. It is their duty to obey and care for the dominant family member—the husband and father.

In the situation with the Martinez couple, duty plays a less prominent role. It is of greater importance that when a family member is ill, love and concern are demonstrated through care and attention. The nurses might have instructed Mrs. Martinez to help her husband in ways that would not hinder his rehabilitation. For example, they could have showed her how to massage lotion onto his hands.

Control may also play a role in the failure to care for oneself. Each of the situations described above involved a man whose culture clearly acknowledged his power and authority. All of these men, however, were reduced to a state of physical weakness by their medical condition. Ordering people around and having them wait upon one's every need are ways of demonstrating dominance. It may masquerade as helplessness, but it is a way of maintaining control.

The hospital staff often has conflicts with family members over issues other than self-care or too many visitors.

Demanding Families

Homa Tehrani, a fifty-year-old widow from the Middle East, was admitted   82 to the stroke unit of the hospital. She was accompanied by several family members, including her son. Although Mrs. Tehrani herself was not a "difficult" patient, her family made things quite difficult for the hospital staff. Her son, Daruish, was the biggest culprit.

First, he demanded that visiting hours (10 A.M. to 8 P.M.) be extended to 7 A.M. to 10 P.M. for his mother, saying that she needed a family member by her side at all times. The hospital complied, even allowing Daruish to sleep in a chair next to his mother's bed.

Next, he demanded that his mother be attended only by females, as is the Muslim custom. Again the hospital complied. He would constantly demand, not ask, that his mother's every need be taken care of immediately. The staff became extremely frustrated. Didn't he realize that they had other patients to care for as well as his mother? Soon everyone came to resent the Tehrani family.

Why were they so demanding? In Middle Eastern culture, the way that family members show their love and concern for their loved ones is to make sure they receive the best care possible. The way to do this is to insist that the staff do their jobs—in fact, do more than their jobs.

As someone who has had family members hospitalized I can well understand the frustration of having someone you care for be seriously ill, yet lacking the medical skills to do anything to help the patient. Staying "on top of" the nurses feels like you're doing something for your loved one. Although this example focuses on a Middle Eastern family, because their culture allows them to be more openly verbally aggressive, families from any ethnic background can be demanding.

What can the staff do? I would suggest:

- At the beginning of the patient's hospitalization, spend a few minutes with the family, asking questions about the patient.
- Show that you care.
- Tell them that you will be happy to talk with them on a regular basis (set up a schedule that you feel comfortable with) so you can update them on the patient's condition and they can share their concerns.

- Give the family small, helpful tasks they can do, such as massaging lotion onto the patient's hands or feet.
- Let them feel they are doing something for the patient.

Often, families become demanding because they feel helpless and out of control; by following these suggestions, you can help to alleviate some of their frustration.

Gifts

83   A more pleasant problem arose during a Korean woman's discharge. Mrs. Chow had been cared for during her week in the hospital by a nurse named Florine. Florine frequently stopped in to see Mrs. Chow, offering to help in any way she could to make her patient more comfortable. Mrs. Chow's family were often there and observed Florine's kindness. When Mrs. Chow was being discharged, her twenty-five year-old son, Jim, took Florine aside and gave her some money. Florine thanked him but refused it, explaining that she could not accept money for doing her job. Furthermore, it was against hospital policy. He insisted that she take it and put it in her pocket. "My mother wants you to have this. She wants to thank you." Florine took the money from her pocket, this time more adamant in her refusal. Jim in turn became extremely embarrassed.

In Korea, it is common for the family to give a patient's nurse food, money, or a special gift to show gratitude for the care she is giving. For Florine to refuse the gift was both insulting and improper. Reciprocity is important in many Asian cultures. When someone does something for another, something is owed in exchange. If the exchange is not completed, the person receiving the kindness is in the other's debt. Since this is an uncomfortable position to be in, it is extremely important not to let such indebtedness occur. A gift to the nurses satisfies the reciprocal obligation.

The stalemate ended when Florine told Jim to take the money and buy some candy for all the nurses to share. This suggestion took care of the Chow family's need to show their appreciation and allowed Florine to adhere to her own values and hospital policy.

The families of Jewish patients also often give nurses gifts while the patient is in the hospital. It is not done so much through a feeling of obligation and reciprocity, however, than as a way of ensuring good care.

Whatever the reason, when a family member presents a gift to the nurse, she will create a great deal of awkwardness if she refuses it. The solution most commonly practiced is for the nurse to share the gift with all the other nurses on the floor.

Family Structure and Kinship

A final family problem involves the issue of who should sign informed consents. Legally, only the parents or legal guardian of a child may sign. In some cultures, however, other persons might be more appropriate—a Navaho boy's grandparent or maternal uncle, for example.

It is not uncommon for Native American grandparents to raise their grandchildren while the parents leave the reservation to work. As the child's primary caretaker, a grandparent might bring a child in to the hospital. Legally, however, the grandparent would not be able to sign a consent form for the child.

The role of the Navaho maternal uncle is a bit more complicated. It is based on the kinship structure of Navaho society. American kinship structure is *bilateral*; we are equally related to members of both sides of our family. Social ties might be closer to one side, but the legal relationship is identical. Many other cultures are *unilineal*, that is, they trace their descent from either a male or a female ancestor. A member of a patrilineal culture (such as many in the Middle East) is considered a member of the father's family, rather than the mother's. In contrast, a member of a matrilineal culture (such as the Navaho or Hopi or some African tribes) is a member of the mother's family, rather than the father's.

Although women tend to have greater power and respect in matrilineal societies than in patrilineal ones, property is passed on from male to male. In matrilineal societies, a boy will inherit from his closest male relative. In this case, it will be his mother's brother, because the boy is not considered a member of his father's family. His father will pass on any property or privileges to his own sister's children. Genetically, this arrangement makes sense. A boy always shares the genes of his mother's brother. It is not so certain that he will carry those of his mother's husband. It is not hard to imagine a situation in which a Navaho man might bring his nephew into the hospital, only to be told he is not empowered to sign an informed consent.

Summary

Family structure and relationships are not the same in every culture. In many cases, accommodation will be difficult, if not impossible, given hospital architecture, American medical values, and the American legal system. At the very least, however, greater understanding of the ways of other cultures may have a positive effect on the attitudes of those providing patient care.

Chapter 7
Men and Women

Sex and gender are frequent sources of conflict and misunderstanding. Not every culture has been affected by the women's movement. Few share the American ideal of equality between the sexes.

Informed Consent

84   A twenty-six-year-old Mexican woman named Rosa Gutierrez brought her two-month-old son to the emergency room. Rosa was concerned because he had diarrhea and had not been nursing. The staff discovered that he was also suffering from sepsis, dehydration, and high fever. The physician wanted to perform a routine spinal tap, but Rosa refused to allow it. When asked why, she said she needed her husband's permission before anything could be done to the baby. The staff tried to convince her that this was a routine procedure, but Rosa was adamant. Nothing could be done until her husband arrived.

Although legally Rosa could have signed the consent, culturally she lacked the authority. In the traditional Mexican household, the man is the head of the family and makes all major decisions. Rosa was unwilling to violate that norm. Fortunately, her husband soon arrived and signed the informed consent.

Women and Authority

85   An Iranian mother and father admitted their thirteen-month-old child, Ali, to the pediatrics unit. After three days of rigorous testing and examination, it was discovered that Ali had Wilms tumor, a type of childhood cancer. Fortunately, the survival rate is 70 to 80 percent with proper treatment.

Before meeting with the pediatric oncologist to discuss Ali's treatment, Mr. and Mrs. Mohar were concerned and frightened, yet cooperative.

Afterward, however, they became completely uncooperative. They refused permission for even the most routine procedures. Mr. Mohar would not even talk with the physician or the nurses. Instead, he called other specialists to discuss Ali's case.

After several frustrating days, the oncologist decided to turn the case over to a colleague. He met with the Mohars and found them extremely cooperative. What caused their sudden reversal in behavior? The fact that the original oncologist was a woman.

Even though the Mohars had described themselves as "Americanized," the Iranian tradition of male authority was still strong. They could not accept a woman making life-and-death decisions for their son. Ali's treatment was too important to be decided by a woman.

Several weeks later, it became necessary to insert a permanent line into Ali to administer his medication. The nurse attempted to show Mrs. Mohar how to care for the intravenous line, but Mr. Mohar stopped her. "It is my responsibility only. You should never expect my wife to care for it." Throughout each encounter with the hospital staff, Mrs. Mohar remained silent. She deferred to her husband.

Interestingly enough, the nurses had few problems with the Mohars. They were treated with respect because, as Mr. Mohar stated, they were functioning under the direction of the physician. Their only problem was in understanding why the Mohars initially refused treatment for Ali. They had assumed that since both parents were educated in American universities and had described themselves as Americanized, they really were. The stress of their son's illness, however, had made them revert to traditional ways. The importance of male dominance in the Middle East is also a major factor in the following situations.

Male Dominance

Nader and Shahab, two healthy looking Iranian men in their late twenties, came into the emergency room demanding to see a doctor. Julie, the nurse on duty, asked what the problem was. Nader curtly responded that he wanted to see a doctor, not a nurse. Julie calmly explained that he first had to be assessed by a nurse. Nader and his friend did not want to wait, however. Julie said they became loud, pushy, and insulting. Roberta, another nurse, came on the scene and told them that Nader did not appear to be seriously ill and would have to be patient. The doctor would see him soon. Nader then stormed past the two nurses, headed into the patient area, and demanded to see a doctor immediately. The nurses had to call security.

What caused Nader's behavior? He felt he warranted the attention of a male doctor, not a mere female nurse. It is common in Iranian culture to want the "top man" in the field. He also probably felt uncomfortable talking with a woman about his problem. He had a venereal disease.

Later, Nader telephoned the emergency room and asked for Julie. "My friend and I have quite a bit of money. Why don't you and another nurse join us?" Needless to say, Julie did not accept his proposition. She was mystified as to what gave him the impression that she would even consider going out with him. Julie had probably made eye contact with Nader, creating the impression that she was sexually "loose" and interested in dating him.

Domineering Husbands

87   A nineteen-year-old Saudi Arabian woman named Sheida Nazih had just given birth. Her husband, Abdul, had been away on business during most of their ten-month marriage but brought her to the United States to have their baby. He moved into the hospital room with Sheida immediately after she gave birth. He kept the door to their room shut and questioned everyone who entered, including the nurses. The nurses were not happy with this procedure but felt they had no choice except to comply.

Although Sheida could speak some English, the only time she would speak directly to the nurses was when Abdul was out of the room. Otherwise, he answered all questions addressed to her. He also decided when she would eat and bathe. As leader of the family, Abdul felt it was his role to act as intermediary between his wife and the world.

Authority Figures in the Family

88   Magdi Bal was a twenty-seven-year-old woman from Saudi Arabia. Her father was at her bedside when Danielle was doing her preoperative assessment. The surgery Magdi was about to undergo could result in sterilization. Danielle wanted to make sure that Magdi understood before signing the consent. The problem was that her father refused to allow her to sign. Mr. Bal was insistent that Magdi not have a hysterectomy under any circumstances.

The staff were outraged. If the surgeon found uterine cancer, as he expected, a hysterectomy might be the only thing that could save Magdi's life. The physician, Dr. Allen, spoke with Magdi. She said that she wanted to leave all decisions to her father. Dr. Allen spoke next with Mr. Bal. He was adamant—no hysterectomy, no matter what. The physician had no choice but to proceed without compromising Magdi's reproductive system.

Danielle spoke with Mr. Bal while Magdi was in surgery. He explained that if Magdi could not bear children, she would not get married. If she could not marry, her worth would be greatly diminished in the eyes of their culture.

Saudi culture is strongly male dominant. It was entirely consistent that an unmarried daughter, even a twenty-seven-year-old one, would let her father make all the decisions. Once she married, her husband would take over that job. Furthermore, it is common in Saudi Arabia for a woman to live with her husband's family after marriage. If Magdi could not marry, she would be a burden to her family for the rest of her life.

The doctors and nurses involved in the case later met to discuss it. All were angry with the father for his apparent lack of concern regarding his daughter's health. The women were particularly angry at Magdi for not being more independent. They were further incensed when Danielle told them what Mr. Bal had said. "We are not baby-making machines and our ability to have a productive life is not dependent on having children!"

Once they had vented their anger, they realized that it was not their place to judge. The patient had maintained her rights—in this case, the right to choose someone else to make the decision. They recognized that their values were different from that of the patient's; in other words, they achieved a measure of cultural relativism.

In the case just described, it was a parent who had authority over an adult child. In the following case, it was the grandparents who were in charge. Tony Romano, the eight-year-old son of Gypsy parents, was afflicted with Guillain-Barré syndrome. He had lost control over all his muscles, including those of his respiratory system. Whenever the male physician asked to speak with the parents, the paternal grandmother and two aunts insisted that he speak with them instead. The grandmother said she did not want the parents to see the child. When the issue of signing informed consent forms came up, the grandmother said they would have to wait until her husband arrived.

Shortly thereafter, a meeting was called with the physician, the two grandfathers, a great-grandfather, and a few uncles. The parents were excluded from the conference by the elder males, who later had the father sign the consent form. The grandmothers were excluded without discussion. It was assumed that only the elder males would take part.

Family members did not allow the Romanos to see their child until two days after his admission, when his condition had stabilized. When his mother finally saw Tony, she became hysterical. The group forbade her to see him again for a while. Family members frequently asked the staff for information about the child's condition, but all decisions were made by Tony's grandfather.

One of the nurses finally asked Tony's grandmother why the boy's parents were not allowed to see him or talk with the physicians. She explained, "They are too young. They are just babies." Tony's father was twenty-eight, his mother twenty-four.

Gypsy marriages are often arranged when the couple are in their mid-teens. After marriage, they usually live with the husband's parents and are sheltered from adult responsibilities and decisions for many years. Wisdom is thought to come with age. The Romanos were still considered children despite the fact that they were parents.

This attitude was very difficult for the nurses to accept. Anglo American culture expects parents to assume full responsibility for their children, no matter what their age. Legal consent for medical procedures may be given only by the parents. Information regarding a child's condition is given only to the parents. In some cases, only the parents are allowed to visit the child. It was very disconcerting for the nurses to have all the rules changed, but the Gypsies insisted on doing things their own way.

The fact that all the important decisions were made by the men, with no input from the women, is also cultural. Gypsies have a male dominated (and age-dominated) society. Women are not allowed to interrupt men's conversations, let alone join them in making decisions.

In general, knowing who holds the position of authority can help resolve difficult situations. Nurses who have worked with Gypsies have said that if they can gain the cooperation of the king, they can maintain some control.

In many cultures, including Gypsy, Asian, Middle Eastern, and Hispanic, males are traditionally the authority figures. Unless they are very Westernized, it is often best to consider them as the spokespersons for the family. They are generally the ones who will make the decisions. This recommendation may be difficult for those with feminist leanings, but it is likely to be the most productive approach. Age is also a sign of authority in Gypsy and Asian cultures so initial conversations should be addressed to the eldest male.

It is unwise, however, to assume that males are always in charge. In matrilineal cultures such as the Navaho, the oldest women may have the greatest authority and decision-making power. The same may be true in many Black families. Although Black Americans are not matrilineal, the structure of the common single-parent family household may lead to the same result.

Preferential Treatment

90   The gender of a child can influence the treatment it receives from the family. A fifteen-year-old Taiwanese boy named Henry Ting was dying of liver cancer. His parents spent as much time with him as possible during

the year he was a patient at the hospital. One of them always spent the night with Henry, even though they had two daughters, aged eleven and thirteen, at home. Henry's mother prepared most of his meals. His father often drove to Chinatown to obtain Chinese herbs they hoped would help his condition. Mr. and Mrs. Ting were extremely devoted parents—at least to their son. The nurses were shocked to hear the Tings state on several occasions that it would have been better if one of their daughters had cancer instead. Did they value their daughters so little?

As discussed in the previous chapter, sons play an important role in traditional Chinese culture. Henry was their first-born and their only son. He would be the one to carry on the family name and care for them in their old age. If he died, whom could they rely on? Who would carry on the Ting name? Henry had always been given preferential treatment. The daughters understood their parents' attitude and did not seem to mind. It was the way things were. They, too, spent all their free time with Henry, catering to his frequent demands.

The nurses had difficulty accepting this situation. They understood the Tings' position intellectually but not emotionally. They responded by frequently pointing out how kind and sweet their daughters were. They also recommended that a psychologist meet with the family. The session was a waste of time. Although polite, the Tings refused to speak openly with the psychologist. In Asian culture, psychotherapy is reserved for the hopelessly mentally insane and carries a great deal of stigma. It is not surprising that they would not speak with him.

After a year in the hospital, Henry died. Two years later, his parents had still not recovered. They visited the cemetery daily. The elder daughter did volunteer work at the hospital to help "pay" for the care Henry received, and the younger daughter planned to join her when she became sixteen.

In a situation such as that involving the Tings, nothing can be done to change the parents' attitudes. Although it may be difficult, nurses should try to understand their point of view. Preference for sons is so strong in some cultures that, according to reports from countries such as China and India, there are many fewer females than would be statistically expected. This is thought to be due to differential care of sick children (i.e., ill sons are taken to the doctor right away; when daughters are sick, parents "wait and see") as well as selective abortion and infanticide.

Female Purity and Modesty

In many parts of the world, female purity and modesty are major values. These can have important repercussions in a health care setting.

A twenty-three-year-old Saudi Arabian woman named Nasrin Hassan was brought into the emergency room by her husband. Stephanie, the nurse on duty, introduced herself and asked Nasrin how she could help her. Her husband, Jamal, answered that she was bleeding and had pain in her lower abdomen. She was three months pregnant. Stephanie told the couple that Nasrin would have to put on a patient gown so the doctor could examine her.

Jamal refused. He would not allow Nasrin to undress, and he certainly would not permit a strange man to examine her. Stephanie and the attending doctor explained that Nasrin was probably having a miscarriage and could bleed to death if she did not receive medical attention. Their arguments were futile. Jamal abruptly left the hospital with his wife still in pain and bleeding vaginally. Later that evening, the Hassans returned. This time, Jamal consented to having his wife transferred to another hospital, where a female doctor could examine and care for her.

92   In a similar case, a twenty-eight-year-old Arab man named Abdul Nazih refused to let a male lab technician enter his wife's room to draw blood. She had just given birth. When the nurse finally convinced Abdul of the need, he reluctantly allowed the technician in the room. He took the precaution, however, of making sure Sheida was completely covered. Only her arm stuck out from beneath the blankets. Abdul watched the technician intently throughout the procedure.

Another time, the toilet in Sheida's room overflowed. Abdul flew into a rage when three men from engineering and housekeeping were about to enter the room after knocking. He refused to allow them in. The toilet went unrepaired until the couple left the next day.

All three incidents stem from the fact that among Arabs family honor is one of the highest values. Since family honor is tied to female purity, extreme modesty and sexual segregation must be maintained at all times. Hospitals that do not have female physicians on staff should have a referral system so one can be found when needed. Female housekeepers should clean the rooms of Middle Eastern females. Male nurses definitely should not be assigned to female Muslim patients. Same-sex staff should be used whenever possible.

Female "Circumcision"

93   An Egyptian woman in labor presented an unusual problem for the nursing staff. Her vagina was severely deformed, and they were unable to find any of the appropriate "landmarks." The entire area appeared to have been badly burned, yet no other parts of her body showed evidence of fire. The doctor and nurses were mystified. They did not realize that the woman had been "circumcised."

One way "female purity" is maintained in the Middle East is by keeping the woman covered and veiled. Another method, used in some remote regions, and particularly in parts of Africa, is "female circumcision" ("female genital mutilation" in the human and women's rights literature). It is believed that the practice reduces women's sexual desire, and that without it, women might be unable to control their exceptionally strong libido, and family honor might be lost.

The procedure is generally performed when a girl is seven or eight years old. Older women will come in the night, hold her down, and then start cutting. The most minor form involves cutting off the tip of the clitoris. The most severe, known as infibulation, is the removal of the entire clitoris, labia minora, and parts of the labia majora. The outer lips of the vagina are then held together with thorns, sutures, or a paste-like material. A small opening is left for urine and menstrual blood. The girl's legs are tied together for several weeks until she heals. As can be imagined, this practice often leads to a myriad urinary, menstrual, and intrapartum problems, apart from the risk of infection and death at the time.

In 1985, a world congress was held in Africa in an effort to reduce or eradicate the practice. Surprisingly, the greatest opposition to the elimination of the custom came not from men but from older women and young girls. The older women wanted to maintain tradition. The young girls were afraid that if they were not circumcised, they would be unable to find husbands. Circumcision is seen as the ultimate proof of purity; why would any boy marry a woman without a guarantee of her virginity? In the years since that world congress little, if any, progress has been made toward eradication of the custom. In fact, newspaper and magazine reports indicate that it is spreading, as African women move out of Africa. Anthropologists recognize that it is difficult, if not impossible, to merely eliminate a traditional cultural ritual; efforts would be better aimed at trying to promote the *sunna* form, which involves cutting only the tip of the clitoris, over infibulation.

Doctors and nurses caring for circumcised women should be especially sensitive to their needs and feelings. Female providers should be used whenever possible, and the patient should be kept draped for privacy. Physicians need to know how to handle labor and delivery, since the episiotomy must be done at an earlier stage. Above all, do not express any ridicule or judgment. You might, however, gently discuss the relationship between their infibulation and any health problems they may have experienced, so that they can make an informed choice for their own daughters. It might also be appropriate to let them know that the practice raises issues of illegality and child abuse in the United States.

Female Virginity

94   The importance of female virginity and purity are unfortunately well illustrated in the following case. Fatima, an eighteen-year-old Bedouin girl from a remote, conservative village, was brought into an American air force hospital in Saudi Arabia after she received a gunshot wound in her pelvis. She had been shot by her cousin Hamid. Her family had arranged for her to marry him, as was local custom, but she wanted nothing to do with him. She was in love with someone else. An argument ensued, and Hamid left. He returned several hours later, drunk, and shot Fatima, leaving her paralyzed from the waist down.

Fatima's parents cared for her for several weeks after the incident but finally brought her to the hospital, looking for a "magic" cure. The physician took a series of x-rays to determine the extent of Fatima's injuries. To his surprise, they revealed that she was pregnant. Sarah, the American nurse on duty, was asked to give her a pelvic exam. She confirmed the report on the x-rays. Fatima, however, had no idea that she was carrying a child. Bedouin girls are not given any sex education.

Three physicians were involved in the case: an American neurosurgeon who had worked in the region for two years; a European obstetrics and gynecology specialist who had lived in the Middle East for ten years; and a young American internist who had recently arrived. No Muslims were involved. The x-ray technician was sworn to secrecy. They all realized they had a potentially explosive situation on their hands. Tribal law punished out-of-wedlock pregnancies with death.

The obstetrician arranged to have Fatima flown to London for a secret abortion. He told the family that the bullet wound was complicated and required the technical skill available in a British hospital.

The only opposition came from the American internist. He felt the family should be told about the girl's condition. The other two physicians explained the seriousness of the situation to him. Girls in Fatima's condition were commonly stoned to death. An out-of-wedlock pregnancy is seen as a direct slur upon the males of the family, particularly the father and brothers, who are charged with protecting her honor. Her misconduct implies that the males did not do their duty. The only way for the family to regain honor is to punish the girl—by death.

Finally, the internist acquiesced and agreed to say nothing. At the last minute, however, the reluctant physician decided he could not live with his conscience. As Fatima was being wheeled to the waiting airplane, he told her father about her pregnancy.

The father did not say a word. He simply grabbed his daughter off the gurney, threw her into the car, and drove away. Two weeks later, the obstetrician saw one of Fatima's brothers. He asked him how Fatima was. The boy looked down at the ground and mumbled, "She died." Family honor had been restored. The ethnocentric internist had a nervous breakdown and had to be sent back to the United States.

Modesty

Modesty is valued in many cultures. Phan Tran, a fifty-seven-year-old Viet-   95
namese woman, was brought into the emergency room by her husband, son, and daughter-in-law. Mrs. Tran had not been eating well for the past month and her fluid intake was poor. A stroke two years earlier had left her paralyzed on the left side. She was rapidly deteriorating, and her family was concerned. The information was conveyed by her son; Mrs. Tran spoke no English.

After examining her, the doctor ordered some tests, along with a Foley catheter and intravenous therapy. Even though she was covered from the waist up, Mrs. Tran was extremely embarrassed when the nurse inserted the catheter. She avoided eye contact and turned her face to the wall. The nurse, sensing her discomfort, did the procedure as quickly as possible.

The area between the waist and knees is considered particularly private by Southeast Asians. Even though Mrs. Tran's upper body was covered, the most intimate part was being exposed. Traditional Asian physicians do not touch a woman's body except to take her pulse. Instead, the woman points to the corresponding area of a doll to indicate the site of her problem. Only a woman's husband should see her genitals.

There is little to be done in such cases other than to respect the patient's modesty and to keep as much of her body covered as possible. Only procedures that are absolutely necessary should be done. Routine pelvic exams, for example, should be avoided.

Sofia Toledo, a sixty-five-year-old upper-class Mexican woman, refused   96
to be dialyzed when she learned that her usual dialysis station was unavailable. She said she would wait until her next treatment, when she could have her customary place. Unfortunately, this was not a viable alternative. Missing a treatment could result in serious complications or even death. When Julia, the nurse, asked her why the new station was unacceptable, Mrs. Toledo was very vague.

Julia finally called Mrs. Toledo's daughter, and together they solved the problem. Mrs. Toledo's usual station was unusual in that it could not be seen very well by the nurses or the patients at the other dialysis stations. The rest of the stations were very open, designed for high visibility by the nurses. To be dialyzed, the patient had to remove her pants and don a patient gown. Her underwear was exposed during the process. Mrs. Toledo's sense of modesty, a quality very strong in Hispanic women, made the more open station intolerable.

Julia said that at the time she found Mrs. Toledo's behavior annoying. She and the other nurses saw it as a delay that would prevent them from leaving early. They did not want to have the extra work of moving machinery or remixing the dialysate. She did not understand the importance of modesty in Hispanic culture, but she did realize that it was important to Mrs. Toledo, a normally compliant patient. In this case, a screen or curtain might have alleviated the problem.

Summary

What conclusions can be drawn from these cases? In general, same-sex physicians and nurses should be assigned if possible when dealing with non-Anglo ethnic groups. Try to keep patients' genitals covered whenever possible. Recognize that sex roles and authority figures vary, though males generally hold the dominant position. Use that knowledge when dealing with patients or families from other ethnic groups. This advice may rankle many women, who may interpret it as reinforcing male domination. Perhaps it does, but if the goals are patient compliance, smooth working relationships, and the best possible patient care, this will be the most expedient way of achieving them.

Chapter 8
Staff Relations

Not only is the patient population culturally diverse, but the staff population is as well. In addition to Anglo staff, hospitals frequently have large populations of doctors from Asia and the Middle East, nurses from the Philippines and Mexico, and orderlies from a variety of countries. This chapter will address some of the problems and misunderstandings that can occur when hospital staff members from diverse cultural backgrounds interact.

Nurses and Doctors

Domineering Doctors

Annie, an American female nurse, had an unpleasant encounter with Dr. Rao, an East Indian male physician. He had ordered her to restrain a patient whom she felt did not need restraining. When she confronted him with her opinion, he became angry and accused her of questioning his authority. When she asked him why he felt the patient needed to be restrained, his only response was, "Because I'm the doctor and I feel that the patient needs to be restrained." Annie was angry at this obvious non-answer. As a nurse, part of her job was to be a patient advocate, and she did not feel that the patient's needs were being met. As their argument continued, an East Indian nurse who had observed the encounter told the physician that this was America and the rules were different here. "This is not India where you can do whatever you want because you men are the only ones who have rights. You need to explain to her why you want the patient restrained, because the patient has rights and the nurse has the right to know why she's restraining the patient."

Upset by the support given Annie, Dr. Rao left the room. The East Indian nurse explained to Annie that his ego was hurt; in India, it is considered highly disrespectful for a nurse to question a doctor. Does this mean that nurses should never question Indian physicians? Obviously not. Perhaps the most effective solution would be to have all foreign health care personnel participate in an in-service seminar on the culture of the American health care system. However, until that happens, since such physicians are not as likely to change their behavior, nurses who want to communicate most effectively with such co-workers might utilize a less confrontational approach.

98   Dr. Fukushima, a Japanese physician, ordered Lisa to give a patient a certain dosage of a medication. Lisa refused on the grounds that the dosage might be harmful to the patient. Dr. Fukushima insisted, but she was adamant. The interesting twist to this situation is that when Dr. Fukushima reported Lisa to her supervisor, he suggested that she should have agreed to give the medication, but simply not have done it.

Asians generally believe it is important both to avoid conflict and to show respect for authority. Rather than refuse directly, it is more appropriate to agree to the supervisor's face and then not follow through. Americans, in contrast, feel it is important to be direct and honest. Disagreement is not avoided. Assertiveness is valued, as is an egalitarian ideal. Dr. Fukushima's major complaint was not that the nurse disobeyed him, but that she disagreed to his face, thereby denying him proper respect.

It would be easy to suggest that nurses dealing with Asian physicians take that advice, but it is not that simple. Laws require nurses to follow through on orders they agree to. Nurses would be well-advised, however, to remember that Asian men are very concerned about their dignity and self-esteem. And, once again, hospitals should consider offering foreign-born physicians training in the role of nurses in American hospitals.

Submissive Nurses

The next incident illustrates the contrast between the attitude that most American nurses have toward physicians and that held by many Asian nurses. It serves as a reminder that arrogance can be found in American-born as well as foreign-born doctors.

99   Janine, an Anglo nurse, and Lourdes, a Filipino nurse, were passing out patients' breakfast trays while the physicians were making rounds. One of the Anglo doctors grabbed a cup of coffee and a carton of milk from a tray. Lourdes rolled her eyes but said nothing. Janine told him the milk and coffee belonged to a patient. He replied that he needed it more than the patient did. Janine persisted. "If you take that, it means that patient doesn't get his morning coffee. Think how you'd feel."

As the angry physician headed down the hall, he deliberately dropped the coffee cup on the floor. Lourdes jumped to get a towel and clean up the mess. Janine stopped her, insisting that the physician clean it up him-self. Lourdes looked at her in shock and replied, "You've got guts!"

Janine responded to the physician's behavior with typical American as-sertiveness. Filipinos are raised to respect authority. Rolling her eyes was her only visible sign of frustration. She was also trying to avoid conflict and maintain harmony, important Asian values.

Filipino respect for authority also helps explain why Perla, another Filipino nurse, took the blame for something that was the doctor's fault. A specialist physician called the intensive care nursery at 6 A.M. and spoke with Perla. He asked why Dr. Michaels, the resident physician, had not included specific medications in a child's treatment. Perla said she would speak to him. She passed on the specialist's recommendations, but Dr. Michaels chose not to act on them. 100

At the shift change, Perla made her report to Roberta, the patient care coordinator, and the incoming nurses. Roberta questioned Dr. Michaels about the medication. Perla interrupted, stating, "It's my fault. I should have thought of that myself. I've checked the orders and the blood work results and I should have considered that." Roberta defended Perla, say-ing it was not her responsibility; she had told Dr. Michaels. It had be-come his responsibility. The resident agreed and absolved Perla of any blame.

Perla later explained to Roberta that she could not let Dr. Michaels take the blame because she did not want to see him "lose face," espe-cially in front of a nurse.

Nurse to Nurse

Gender Role Conflict

Traditional dominant and subordinate roles can also create friction among hospital staff. For example, Ikem Nwoye, the Nigerian male nurse assistant discussed in Chapter 2, would have what one nurse described as a temper tantrum whenever a female registered nurse asked him to do something. Other times he would sulk and simply leave the room. What he would not do is take instructions from a woman. In Nigeria, men are considered superior to women. Men tell women what to do, not the reverse. 101

Nursing is a hierarchical profession in which orders are followed ac-cording to rank, not sex. The nurses thus expected the nurse assistant to do what they told him. As a Nigerian male, Ikem felt that he should not have to take directions from females, despite his lower professional rank-ing. Unless someone with this cultural disposition can be placed under the supervision of another man, it will be difficult to maintain a viable working relationship on the floor.

The Role of the Nurse

102   Josepha DeLeon, a Filipino nurse, did not get along well with her co-workers. The nursing staff on her unit was composed of two Anglo Americans, two Nigerians, and Josepha. She felt her co-workers were taking advantage of her, since they would ask for assistance whenever they saw her. Josepha was angry over what she perceived as obvious discrimination. She cheered herself by reminding herself that she was a better nurse than the others; she could do her work without their help. In addition, she was not lazy like they were. She took care of her patients; the other nurses insisted that their patients take care of themselves.

One day, Rena, one of the Anglo nurses, was unusually friendly, so Josepha opened up to her. As they got to know each other better, Josepha shared her feelings of being taken advantage of. Rena explained that it was common procedure for the nurses to help each other with their work. Rena confided that the others thought Josepha was being snobbish and proud because she never asked for help. What Josepha had interpreted as laziness on the part of the others was seen by them as being team players. Rena also explained that American health care providers believe that independence is important and encourage self-care among their patients.

Josepha was stunned by Rena's revelations. Rena offered to help bridge the communication gap between Rena and her co-workers. Rena explained to the others that Josepha was trying to save face by never asking for help; she didn't want them to think she couldn't do her job. Josepha began to teach her patients self-care and to ask her co-workers for assistance. Over time, the cross-cultural misunderstandings were resolved, and Josepha's co-workers became her best friends.

103   Vuong Hue disliked her job as a nurse when she first arrived in America from Vietnam. Before fleeing her native country for her life, she had been happy in her nursing position. However, as she soon learned, nursing in America was far different from that in Vietnam. American nurses had four roles: to provide professional technical care; to provide nonspecialized care (e.g., bathing patients); to serve as patient advocate; and to provide psychosocial nursing. In Vietnam, she had but one function—to provide professional technical care. Her co-workers thought she was stuck-up because she acted as if bathing patients and cleaning bedpans were beneath her dignity. It wasn't that, exactly; she just wasn't used to having to do it. As any American-trained nurse will admit, that is not the most pleasant part of the job! Psychosocial nursing

was unnecessary as well; more than that, Hue viewed it as improper. The patient's family took care of personal issues; it was rude for her to pry into their personal lives.

It took Hue several years, but she eventually became accustomed to the different roles that American nurses must take. Her co-workers no longer saw her as stuck-up. It might be helpful for American hospitals to have special in-service programs for foreign nurses to discuss explicitly the differences in nursing roles in various cultures. It would go a long way to avoiding misunderstanding.

Leadership

Problems also arise from the traditionally passive female roles valued in most Asian cultures. Myung Soon Park, a Korean charge nurse in intensive coronary care, was an excellent worker. She was quiet, industrious, and knowledgeable. She gave the patients good care and was proficient in using the specialized equipment in the unit. In her role as charge nurse, however, Myung Soon was perceived as incompetent. She was unable to lead. She did not offer strong guidance to her staff. She did not counsel or reprimand them. She was indecisive and became apologetic when anyone made a mistake.

Although Myung Soon's personality was partly to blame, her submissiveness was consistent with the traditional role of Korean women. Korean culture is hierarchical, and the ideal woman is passive and subservient. She is taught to avoid conflict and maintain harmony. These values made it difficult for Myung Soon to perform the functions of a good charge nurse. Her co-workers liked her personally but were frustrated by her professional performance.

Myung Soon was aware of the problems she was having. Counseling helped her to realize she could not handle her job. She resigned as charge nurse but continued on as a staff nurse.

Passive Versus Assertive Behavior

A few examples have been given of the passive, submissive behavior of Filipino and other Asian nurses. Many other nurses, however, report the complete opposite. They say that Filipino nurses, for example, can be very assertive, to the point of aggressiveness. What accounts for this discrepancy?

As in any culture, people are born with personality traits that fall along a continuum. Different cultures, however, value and reinforce different aspects of the continuum. If a child is by nature passive and the culture reinforces passivity, socialization will be easy. If the child is by nature as-

104

sertive, socialization will be difficult, but possible. If when that child grows up, he or she moves to a country where assertiveness is valued, years of socialization to be passive may be suddenly undone, as that individual's true nature comes through. The assertiveness may even be exaggerated as a result of years of repression.

Thus, passive Filipino nurses are the ones who were by nature passive even before being socialized in that direction. It will be very difficult to train them to be assertive. The aggressive ones are most likely those who were socialized to be passive against their inherent nature and who now have cultural (American) permission to be assertive.

The Role of the Doctor

105   A cross-cultural misunderstanding between a Middle Eastern male physician and an Anglo American female patient sheds interesting light both on the role of men and women in Middle Eastern culture and the roles of doctors and patients.

Roberta Hansen had been admitted for pneumonia. Abbas Mehraban had been called in to consult when her own physician found some lab results which he could not explain. Dr. Mehraban questioned Roberta about her symptoms, and then told her how he was going to treat her condition. He neither explained his rationale nor included her in the decision-making process. When Roberta tried to question him about her treatment, he gave her only vague responses. Roberta became increasingly angry and yelled at him, using profanity. Her behavior angered the physician so much that he resigned from the case.

Most Americans can probably understand why Roberta was angry, but what about Dr. Mehraban? In the Middle East, doctors are seen as authority figures, and their decisions are not to be questioned. Roberta breached proper Middle Eastern etiquette regarding patient and physician roles. Dr. Mehraban needed some teaching on the relationship between American patients and their physicians, including the patient's "right to know."

Although by American standards, Dr. Mehraban would not be considered a "good" doctor, there are others in which he would. In many Native American and Asian cultures, a "good" doctor does not need to ask the patients a lot of questions. The doctor should be able to diagnose the patient by reading the proper signs. This is in direct conflict with the American approach, which values physicians who *ask* their patients a lot of questions and *listen* to the responses. "Good" American doctors may thus unwittingly lose the respect of some their patients. Perhaps they might judiciously choose to have the nurse ask questions of the patient before they begin their examination.

The American legal and medical systems recognize patients' right to know all the details of their condition. The high incidence of medical malpractice suits also dictates that physicians share all possible complications of any surgical procedure or medication. Such openness and honesty can have a negative effect when dealing with patients from other ethnic groups.

In China and Japan, where doctors are seen as authority figures in a hierarchical and patriarchal society, patients are told little about their condition. Lawsuits are extremely rare. The physician is expected to know best and to use good judgment. If the patient has cancer, the family might be told, but the patient is rarely given the diagnosis. Asians have a tremendous fear of cancer, perceiving it as a death sentence, even though many forms can be successfully treated. Patients told they have cancer often mistakenly assume the situation is hopeless and give up. Loss of will to live can lead to premature death.

Imagine the situation of a Chinese or Japanese patient new to the United States who is told he or she has cancer. The physician may believe it is easily treatable through a combination of surgery, radiation, and chemotherapy. The patient, knowing that doctors never reveal a diagnosis of cancer to a patient, assumes the worst. He or she is going to die immediately. The psychological ramifications can be devastating.

In such a case, it might be advisable to use a technical medical term other than cancer and begin by emphasizing the success of treatment.

Language and Communication Problems

Speaking in the Native Language in the Workplace

One of the problems that comes up most frequently when I do workshops is that of nurses speaking their native languages in the hospital. This is a very interesting issue, with legitimate explanations on both sides.

106

The American nurses dislike it when co-workers speak in their native language for a number of reasons. Most importantly, when, for example, a Filipino nurse speaks to a co-worker in Tagalog in front of a patient, the patient naturally assumes they are talking about him or her. Bilingual parents often speak to each other in a language children don't know when they want to hide something from them. And the news must be bad, otherwise, why would they speak in a foreign language? This can be extremely distressing for the patient and family, and really should be avoided.

It is less critical, but still hurtful, when nurses speak in their native tongues around other employees. American nurses frequently report feeling left out when they walk into a room and several Filipinos continue to converse in Tagalog. They see it as extremely rude.

When this issue comes up in groups, I usually ask the Filipinos to explain why they speak in Tagalog at work, even though they can speak English. Some of their answers are to be expected; others are surprising. Among the expected answers: Away from their native land, it brings them a sense of home and belonging. As one Filipino stated, "Speaking our own language reassures Filipinos that even though we are here in the United States, we still have something that bonds us together, something that we have in common that gives a sense of belonging." In an emergency situation, they feel they can communicate more quickly in their native tongue. Some things, like jokes, do not hold up in translation. They may be embarrassed by their thick accent in English.

I've heard two other explanations which were less predictable. One is that in Filipino culture it is important to show respect to your superiors in the hierarchy—for example, anyone who is older than you. Tagalog has different words which do this; English does not. It could therefore be seen as rude for a Filipino to talk to an elder in English. Another explanation has to do with the fact that, in the Philippines, speaking English is associated with higher social status. If you are Filipino and speak to another Filipino in English, you will be seen as conceited, as acting as though you are better than the other person.

It is important for native English speakers to realize that Filipinos are not intending to be rude when they speak in Tagalog in the presence of others. But Filipinos must also realize that it can be very distressing to patients and can make non-Filipino co-workers feel excluded. Open discussion of all perspectives is usually quite effective. The most equitable solution is to allow hospital employees to speak in their native tongues when on break, as long as no one else is around. When nonspeakers enter the room, they should immediately switch to English. Under no circumstances, however, should they converse in anything other than English around patients (unless, of course, the patient is fluent in that language).

When Emotions Are Controlled Too Well

107   Eva, a Chinese nurse, was caring for a young girl. Eva had been directed by the intern to keep her under close observation due to the fact that she was becoming diaphoretic and pale. After two hours, these conditions continued to worsen, and she was breathing abnormally. Eva was alarmed, but tried to stay calm and composed when she called the patient's doctor. The physician was unavailable, so she spoke to his associ-

ate. She said, "The patient is looking dusky. Can someone come to look at this patient?"

Three minutes passed, and the patient's condition had worsened, yet none of the doctors had arrived. Eva eventually had to call a "code" over the phone, which summoned every doctor at once.

Afterward, Eva was chided by her nurse manager for not indicating the seriousness of the patient's condition when she called the doctor. She should have used the word "now" emphatically, and conveyed a sense of emergency by her tone of voice.

Eva was offended at first, but then realized it was a cultural problem. As a Chinese woman, she had been raised to control her emotions and to remain calm in an emergency. Since that incident, she has learned to employ more "American" communication skills and call for help more assertively when necessary.

When "Yes, I Understand" Means "No, I Don't"

Marsha, an Anglo nurse, attempted to assess the knowledge and technical skills of the critical care nurses in her hospital. Most were from China, Laos, Korea, Vietnam, and the Philippines. The first phase of testing involved a written exam focusing on general principles. Confusion reigned, and the scores were low. Thinking the problem lay in the language of the test, Marsha rewrote the exam. In the new version, the nurses had only to answer yes or no to questions about their knowledge of a specific procedure (e.g., "I understand the principles of hemodynamic monitoring"). Over 90 percent of the questions received a "yes" response. Disturbed by the contradictory results of the two tests, Marsha interviewed several of the test-takers, asking open-ended questions which required them to demonstrate their knowledge. Although their English was proficient, many were unable to answer correctly. Why did they say they understood procedures and principles they clearly did not?

Recall the discussion in Chapter 2, "When 'Yes' May Mean 'No'." The Asian nurses were probably too embarrassed to admit they did not know something. Education is highly valued, and a lack of knowledge indicates a lack of education. The result is a loss of self-esteem. The lesson here is the same as earlier—try to avoid asking yes or no questions. Ask that people *demonstrate* their knowledge instead.

"Please" and "Thank You"

Patty, an Anglo nurse, had been working with Maria, a Korean nurse, for two years. Their relationship had been rather hostile. Patty felt that Ma-

108

109

ria was a very bossy person, never saying "please" or "thank you." She was also perceived as rather cold and stand-offish, as evidenced by the fact that she would rarely call her co-workers by their first name, especially the older ones, even after being asked to do so. Patty decided to interview Maria for a class assignment in order to understand her better.

When discussing her values, Maria explained the importance of respect in Korean culture. People will call each other by their last names, and use special terms when addressing people older than themselves. However the hierarchy works two ways. When asking something of someone younger than yourself, it is unnecessary to say things like, "please," and "thank you," since you are in the higher position and can act more informally. The respect is understood. Since Maria was older than many of the other nurses, she rarely said "please" or "thank you," assuming it was understood. It wasn't; the others merely thought she was rude.

After the interview, Patty realized that her impression of Maria had been totally wrong, and they soon became friends. Nurses must recognize that what is polite in one culture may be seen as rude in another. Open discussion of cultural differences, however, can help alleviate such problems, as it did in the case of Patty and Maria.

"Don't Be Crazy"

110   Another incident with a linguistic basis involved an Anglo nurse who was in the habit of helping out nurses' aides when her own work was done. All the aides but one accepted Sylvia's assistance gratefully. When Sylvia offered to help Celina, a Filipino aide, with the difficult care of her quadriplegic and stroke patients, she declined. Celina was insulted, because in the hierarchical culture in which she had been raised, a supervisor would only offer to help if she felt the worker could not do her job properly. Sylvia responded, "Don't be silly! It's crazy to do this alone. You could get a bad back." Celina took the words "silly" and "crazy" literally to mean that Sylvia thought she was mentally ill, a condition that is highly stigmatized in Filipino culture. No wonder she was insulted. Celina also interpreted the original offer of help to mean that Sylvia thought she was slow and incompetent. Her *amor proprio* (self-esteem) had been wounded.

Sylvia learned of Celina's reaction from another Filipino aide. Celina had not said anything directly to Sylvia because she wanted to avoid conflict and show respect for authority—important values in the Filipino culture. Although Sylvia had, at first, perceived this as "going behind her back," she later learned that the use of a third party go-between is common in many Asian cultures. The next time Sylvia saw Celina, she apologized, saying that she had not understood how Celina felt. Celina explained that she had been raised with certain ideas and was having trouble adjusting to American ways. For example, Filipino nurses feel they have failed if they do not complete all their work on an eight-hour shift. American nurses will simply tell those on the next shift that they were very busy and could not finish everything. By the end of their discussion, Celina and Sylvia came to an understanding and never had any more problems. It is important to realize that words and actions can carry greater significance than we might intend.

Religious Conflicts

Medical personnel also face conflicts between their duty to patients and their own religious beliefs. In one instance, a nurse of the Jehovah's Witness faith was temporarily transferred to the intensive care unit, where she admitted a patient with gastrointestinal bleeding. He required several units of blood. The nurse refused to hang the blood. It was against her religious beliefs even to participate in a blood transfusion. Reluctantly, she did agree to watch it infuse after someone else started it.   111

Carmen, a Filipino nurse, was informed that she was to be the circulating nurse on a therapeutic abortion. She immediately began to cry and told her supervisor that she would leave work unless her assignment was changed. Carmen was a devout Catholic and refused to participate in an abortion. Joyce, her supervisor, was upset. Other Catholic nurses had worked on abortions before. Besides, she was short of personnel and cases were already running over schedule. Joyce agreed to find someone else to circulate, but she asked Carmen to gather the equipment and supplies for the case. Even this was a problem. "If I set down the room, it's just the same as if I were doing the case," she explained. "I have assisted or aided in taking a life." Joyce finally changed her assignment, but not without some resentment.   112

It is often very difficult for people to understand others' religious practices, especially when they cause inconvenience. But it is best, whenever possible, to avoid giving assignments that conflict with individuals' religious convictions. Jehovah's Witness nurses, for example, can be assigned to coronary care or well-baby units, where there is rarely a need to hang blood. Nurses assigned occasional duties that conflict with their religious beliefs can arrange to switch tasks with a co-worker. If their beliefs get in the way of their job too often, however, they should be advised to look for a new job.

Summary

Given the vast cultural diversity of the health care staff in American hospitals, it is sometimes surprising that more conflicts do not occur. The major problems seem to stem from the different roles that doctors and nurses are assigned in different cultures. These are often accentuated by gender role differences. Thus, male physicians from male-dominated countries tend to be even more domineering than American male doctors, and female nurses from such countries tend to be more submissive than American nurses. Rules of polite behavior vary cross-culturally, and are often a source of misunderstanding.

Since rules of behavior are rarely made as explicit as rules of grammar or of the road, conflicts and misunderstanding abound. In most cases, such problems can be avoided or resolved through cultural education. Doctors and nurses from foreign countries could be required to participate in an in-service on the culture of the American hospital system. In addition, workshops in which staff are led to discuss the way things are done in their culture, in which participants can feel free to ask questions and share their feelings, are often successful in alleviating conflicts and misunderstandings.

Chapter 9
Birth

Increasingly, people enter the world in a hospital. Birth is an emotional and generally painful occasion imbued with cultural ritual—and thus, once again, we find the potential for misunderstanding and conflict.

Preparation

Confusion can begin before a woman enters the labor and delivery rooms. In one case, a nurse named Judith came to "prep" an Iranian woman and was surprised to find her pubic area already completely shaved. American women are usually uncomfortable about being shaved in the pubic area and require constant reassurance that more hair is not being shaved off than necessary. For this reason, nurses pride themselves on shaving off the minimal amount of pubic hair necessary for delivery.

Jasmine, an Americanized Iranian woman, later explained to Judith that many Iranian women completely shave their bodies in preparation for both their wedding night and the birth of their children.

Judith reflected upon her own discomfort when others saw her normally clean-shaven legs covered with stubble. She also realized that the Iranian practice made her job easier. These two thoughts helped her view the situation with cultural relativism rather than with ethnocentrism.

Prenatal Care

A common complaint of labor and delivery nurses is that many women do not seek prenatal care. Although this can sometimes result in problems, the primary difficulty is a conflict in perception. Americans are raised to see pregnancy and birth as medical conditions; births usually occur in hospitals under the supervision of doctors. Medical culture also values education (thus, childbirth classes) and a future time orientation (preparation for the coming birth). Prenatal care is an essential part of this package. On the other hand, many Mexican women, for example, view pregnancy as a normal condition, not necessarily requiring the assistance of a physician. Elder women provide the support and information needed. Time orientation is focused on the present rather than the future; hence a frequent lack of prenatal care. Although health care professionals should strive not to impose their values upon their patients, if a woman who has just given birth can be predicted to have high risk pregnancies in the future, health care providers should take the time to explain why prenatal care will be important next time.

Labor Pains

Individuals respond differently to pain, although cultural norms often dictate how it is expressed. This holds true for the pains of labor.

114
    Doris, a Black American, and Miguela, a Filipino, were delivering their babies at the same time. Miguela's contractions were very strong and closely spaced. The baby was positioned a little too high, and there was some discussion of a possible c-section. Despite her difficulties, Miguela cooperated with the doctor's instructions and labored in silence. The only signs of pain or discomfort were her look of concentration and her white knuckles.

In contrast, Doris lay in the delivery room across the hall, moaning and groaning. Although the delivery was progressing normally, her cries increased in intensity. Finally, her bloodcurdling yells resounded through the halls. The hospital personnel compared Doris's behavior to Miguela's and naturally rated it unfavorably. Why was Doris acting like such a baby? Why couldn't she control herself as Miguela did?

Cultural differences account for the behavioral differences. Miguela's culture values stoicism; Doris's culture does not. Filipinos believe that a woman must experience pain and discomfort as a part of childbirth. To express these feelings, however, brings shame upon her. This is true in most Asian cultures.

The culture of American Blacks does not place such restrictions upon its women. Varied emotional expression has always been a part of Black culture. Doris was culturally normal in expressing her pain. Another Black woman might have suffered in silence and still have been culturally normal.

Mexican women are notorious for loud behavior during labor and delivery. It is often possible to identify a Mexican woman in labor simply from the *"aye yie yies"* emanating from her room. Although this chant can be annoying to nurses and patients alike, it is actually a form of "folk Lamaze." To repeat *"aye yie yie"* several times in succession requires long, slow, deep breaths. *"Aye yie yie"* is not just an expression of pain; it is a culturally appropriate method of relieving pain.

Women from some cultures may profit greatly from emphasizing their pain during childbirth. A labor and delivery nurse reported that the most difficult patient she ever attended was Robabeh, an Iranian woman, who yelled and screamed for the entire duration of her labor. After she delivered their child, Robabeh's husband presented her with a three-karat diamond ring. When her nurse commented on the expensive gift, Robabeh responded dramatically, "Of course. He made me suffer so much!" Iranian custom is to compensate a woman for her suffering during childbirth by giving her gifts. The greater the suffering, the more expensive the gifts she will receive, especially if she delivers a boy. Her cries indicate how much she is suffering.

American nurses value cooperation; a cooperative patient is one who is stoic and follows directions. Uncooperative patients, like Robabeh, are often avoided. How can hospital personnel deal with the variety of expressions of women's pain during labor and delivery? As one nurse put it, there are techniques for controlling pain that are more effective than yelling, but the delivery table is hardly the place to educate women in coping skills. If nurses understand why patients behave the way they do, however, they can be more supportive.

As for the patients themselves, it might be very disconcerting for an Asian woman accustomed to controlling her emotions to labor next to a highly expressive Mexican or Middle Eastern woman. Ideally, women might be placed in rooms with women from cultures similar to theirs. Unfortunately, this is not always possible. Sometimes, a brief explanation of cultural differences in the expression of pain might help, particularly a first-time mother who is laboring next to a woman from a more expressive culture.

Labor Attendants

It is currently standard American practice for a woman's husband to assist her in labor and in the delivery of their child. Husbands are expected to be helpful and to attend to their wives' needs. Unfortunately, things do not always work out this way.

Naomi, an Orthodox Jewish woman, was in labor with her third child. She had severe pains, which were alleviated only by back rubs between contractions. Her husband, Aaron, asked Marge, a nurse, to remain in the room to rub Naomi's back. Because she had two other patients to care for, Marge began to instruct Aaron on how to massage his wife. To Marge's surprise, he immediately interrupted her, explaining that he could not touch his wife because she was unclean. Marge, assuming he meant Naomi was sweaty from labor, suggested that he massage her through the sheets. In an annoyed tone, Aaron again explained that he could not touch his wife because she was unclean. He then left the room.

Marge later learned from Naomi that "unclean" referred to a spiritual, rather than a physical, condition. According to the Orthodox Jewish tradition, the blood of both menstruation and birth render a woman unclean and her husband is forbidden to touch her during those times.

Labor and delivery nurses must do everything for the Orthodox Jewish patient whose husband will not participate. This often generates resentment toward both the patient and her husband. Nurses sometimes try to avoid being assigned to Orthodox patients or assign another Jewish nurse to attend to them. As always, a good solution is education. If nurses understand why an Orthodox husband cannot get involved in his wife's labor, they may be more accepting.

117   An Arab husband can be similarly unhelpful during his wife's labor and delivery. After his wife, Azar, was admitted to the unit, Ahmed told the nurse that he would wait outside. Realizing that her patient did not speak English, she asked Ahmed to stay and act as translator. At first, he refused, insisting that it was a woman's place to help in birthing, not a man's. Since there were no Arab women available to translate, however, he reluctantly agreed to stay.

During her entire labor, Ahmed ignored Azar except to translate as requested. She was obviously having a difficult time, expressing her pain quite loudly, but he did nothing to comfort her. The staff grew angry with him. It was inadvisable to insist that Ahmed stay with Azar during childbirth. Because it was inappropriate for him to be there, he felt extremely uncomfortable and did little to help her situation.

Some nurses have reported that Middle Eastern men often do accompany their wives or sisters in the delivery room, but not to assist her. Rather, they are there to "protect" her virtue.

118   A similar case involved a young Mexican couple. Judging from her *"aye yie yies,"* Juanita was in a great deal of pain. When the nurse insisted that her husband, Carlos, attend to her, he very reluctantly entered the room. Rather than help soothe Juanita by holding her hand, speaking gently to her, or wiping her brow, he stood in the corner. He looked up, down, everywhere but at her. The nurse became very angry. She felt that because Carlos had gotten Juanita into this position in the first place, he should be willing to comfort her.

119   In another instance, a Mexican woman named Carmelita had recently moved to California. She was five months pregnant when she began to bleed vaginally. Her mother and husband brought her to the emergency

room, and it became clear that a premature delivery was inevitable. Labor lasted one and a half hours. During this time, Carmelita continuously cried out for her mother. The nursing staff brought her husband into the room to provide moral support, but Carmelita ignored him. He, in turn, sat in a chair a few feet from her bed with his back to her and stared out the door. Carmelita continued to cry for her mother.

In Mexico, it is inappropriate for a husband to attend his wife during delivery. It is a woman's job—ideally the job of her mother. This may be related to the extreme modesty of Mexican women. American nurses who have difficulty believing that the modesty of traditional Mexican women can extend to her own husband should be told of the eighty-five-year-old Mexican woman with a tattoo of a small cross on her upper thigh. No one in her family—including husband and daughters—had ever seen it. She told the nurse who was caring for her that she had done it in her wild and crazy youth.

Whatever the reason, a number of cultural traditions dictate that a husband not see his wife or child until the delivery is over and both have been cleaned and dressed. For those who find these cultural practices hard to understand, consider suddenly being forced to watch one's parents have sex. How would we feel? Would we stand there and coach them? Wipe their sweaty brows? Or would we stand in a corner, looking up, down, everywhere but at them? Sexual relations occur in the presence of children in some parts of the world but are taboo in American culture, just as it is taboo for a Mexican man to watch his wife give birth, though it is a common practice for American men. Younger, more Americanized Mexican couples may want to participate in the delivery process together, but it should not be assumed that the husband is the proper person to coach his wife in this situation.

In the case of the Mexican woman who delivered prematurely, the doctor and nurses involved judged the patient as immature and her husband as unsupportive and ineffective. One of the nurses later suggested that the staff purposely excluded the patient's mother from the delivery room to punish Carmelita for her "immature, inappropriate" behavior. Since the rules allowed only one visitor at a time, the husband's presence prevented Carmelita's mother from attending her daughter. The nurses apparently felt it was her husband's job, and he would attend her or no one would.

In general, Hispanic women prefer that their mothers attend them in labor. This is also true of Asian women, although sometimes the mother-in-law is considered more appropriate. A Korean nurse shared this information in class one day, to the general shock and horror of the rest of the class. As she explained, traditionally, when a Korean woman marries, she goes to live with her husband's parents and spends much of her married life taking care of the needs of her in-laws. This is reversed during childbirth. Then, a mother-in-law must attend to the needs of her daughter-in-law, both during delivery and throughout the month long lying-in period.

Cesarean Section

121   Chue Hong, a Hmong refugee woman, was pregnant with twins. Early in labor, it was discovered that the second twin was lying across the uterus rather than head down. The attending physician recommended a cesarean section. The woman's husband and mother refused, stating their fear that she would die during surgery. Although the doctors and nurses continued to try to persuade the patient and her family that she should consent to the surgical delivery, they remained adamantly against it. As a result, the first twin was delivered without problem but the second twin died. The next morning, the husband returned and requested the placentas, explaining that they had to be separated in order to protect the live infant from death.

Why was the family so opposed to a cesarean section? Perhaps because, like many non-Christian rural Southeast Asians, they feared that souls are attached to different parts of the body. During surgery, they can leave the body, causing illness or death. In such a situation, there is little that the health care team can do except respect the wishes of the patient and family. This case resulted from a conflict in beliefs, and, in America, the patient has the right to refuse medical care.

Post-Partum Lying In

122   Mei-Li, a Chinese woman in her mid-twenties, had just given birth. The hospital staff became concerned when she would neither eat the hospital food nor bathe. Her only nourishment came from the food brought in by her family. Later Mei-Li explained that custom prevented her from bathing for seven days after childbirth and permitted her to eat only certain foods.

123   The following cases also illustrate how Asian cultural practices may result in behavior regarded as odd or unhealthy by Westerners. A twenty-eight-year-old Vietnamese woman named Hanh Ly gave birth to her first child by cesarean section. After the delivery, she requested ice water. Her mother emphatically refused, insisting that she be given hot water to drink instead. After a discussion in Vietnamese, the patient compromised and asked for a pitcher of warm water. The nurse noted that despite the warm temperature, Hanh Ly wore socks and spread a robe over the sheets. When asked if she was cold, she said no.

Su Yong, a nineteen-year-old Vietnamese woman, returned to the hospital with a high fever and abdominal pain twelve days after giving birth. During her stay, she rejected most of the food and liquids prepared by the hospital, refused to shower or wash her hair (despite increasingly strong body odor), and would not get out of bed except to use the bathroom. When she insisted on mounds of blankets in spite of her high temperature and sweating, the nurses feared for her health. 124

A thirty-four-year-old Filipino woman named Flores gave birth via c-section. On the following day, her nurse prepared to bathe her, but she refused. The day after that, the nurse brought Flores a basin of water and a sponge so she could bathe herself. Several hours later, the water was still clean and the towels untouched. When questioned, Flores explained that it was the custom in her culture to refrain from bathing or showering for ten days after giving birth. 125

The patients described above were all practicing versions of the traditional lying-in period observed throughout much of Asia and Latin America. For a period of time after a woman gives birth, her body is thought to be weak and especially susceptible to outside forces. The new mother is encouraged to avoid both exercise and bathing. These traditional practices come into direct conflict with Western health care, which promotes exercise and bathing for new mothers as soon as possible following childbirth.

The traditional practice in China is called "doing the month." It is important to keep the room warm, lest cold or wind enter the new mother's joints. Bathing is considered dangerous for similar reasons. No matter how hot the weather, the traditional Chinese woman will want the windows closed and the air conditioning off.

In Asia, health is believed to depend upon keeping the body in a state of balance. Pregnancy is generally thought to be a hot condition. Giving birth causes the sudden loss of *yang*, or heat, which must be restored. The most effective way to do this is to eat yang foods, such as chicken. Cold liquids should be avoided lest the system receive too great a shock.

Traditional Asian thought has it that the price for not "doing the month" is aches, pains, arthritis, and other ailments when one is old. Although practical circumstances may prevent a woman from observing the entire month, many want to practice at least a shortened version of it. This explains why the patients in the cases described above refused ice water in preference for hot, rejected bathing or exercise, insisted upon keeping extremely warm, and ate only certain foods.

In Mexico the lying-in period lasts for six weeks, the time believed necessary for the womb to return to normal. (In fact, forty-two days is generally the amount of time it takes for the uterus to return to its pre-

pregnant size.) The customs involved are essentially identical to those of the Asian practice: the woman is to rest, stay very warm, and avoid bathing and exercise. Special foods designed to restore warmth to the body are prescribed. Disregarding these practices is believed to lead to aches and pains in later life.

Another problem nurses encounter during the post-partum period involves Pakistani women. It is traditional for them to have a female companion who does everything for the woman—feeding her, hair care, pouring beverages, and all infant care except breastfeeding. If there is no one available to do that for her, a Pakistani woman may expect the nurse to fill that role. This can lead to anger on the part of nurses, who tend to see such patients as demanding and lazy. Instead, they should realize that it is simply the way traditional Pakistani women have been raised to behave after childbirth. They may not know it is done differently in this country.

There are three additional points to be made about the post-partum lying-in period. First, it is designed to give a woman a period of rest between childbirth and returning to work. The women who practice this custom are usually Asian and Latin American. In these cultures women traditionally did not return to office work, but to physical labor in the fields. Because they usually had large families, it might be the only time they had to rest.

Second, avoidance of bathing may also have practical origins. In many countries the water is impure and filled with harmful bacteria. Bathing could introduce these organisms into the body and cause illness. Although conditions in the United States are different, the custom continues.

The third point involves the ways in which different generations adhere to customs. As with Hanh Ly, the Vietnamese woman who wanted ice water but was advised by her mother to drink hot water instead, daughters may be less interested in following traditional customs than their mothers. To avoid her mother's nagging, the daughter may comply with the cultural traditions when the mother is present. When the patient is alone, a nurse may suggest bathing, exercise, and so forth.

Compromises can be made. Although it is important for a patient to drink fluids after childbirth, both hot tea and hot water with lemon deliver the same amount of liquid as ice water without violating custom. Using boiled water (cooled down) may make a sponge bath more acceptable. (This was done in China to remove impurities.) The patient should be kept covered and given socks or slippers to walk in. It is important to explain the reason for bathing and exercise and not to assume that the patient will follow orders that violate the traditions and wisdom of her own culture.

Bonding

Maternal-infant bonding has become a major concern of Western health care professionals in recent decades. Poor bonding has been associated with failure to thrive, child abuse, and psychological problems. It is therefore not surprising that doctors and nurses become concerned when they observe cultural beliefs and practices that appear to reflect poor bonding. They often do not. An example is the case of Thanh Vo, a Vietnamese woman who came to the hospital to deliver her fifth child. After giving birth to a son, she refused to cuddle him, although she willingly provided minimal care such as feeding and changing his diaper. The nursery nurse, feeling sorry for the "neglected" baby, picked him up, cuddled him, and stroked the top of his head. Mrs. Vo and her husband became visibly upset. The baby, who had jaundice, had to remain in the hospital for several days after Mrs. Vo went home. She did not visit her baby even once during the time he remained in the hospital.

126

In the past, nurses who worked in areas with a large Vietnamese population often referred these mothers to social services. Eventually, however, they came to understand that the apparently neglectful behavior did not indicate poor bonding, but instead reflected cultural belief and traditions.

Many people in the more rural areas of Vietnam believe in spirits. Since spirits are particularly attracted to infants and likely to "steal" them (by inducing death), it is important that parents do everything possible to avoid attracting attention to their newborn. For this reason, infants are not verbally fussed over. They are sometimes even dressed in old clothes to "fool" the spirits. The apparent lack of interest new parents demonstrate reflects an intense love and concern for the child, rather than the opposite.

Mrs. Vo and her husband were probably distressed over the nurse's attention to their baby for two reasons. First, they may have feared having attention drawn to their baby. Second, Southeast Asians view the head as private and personal. It is also seen as the seat of the soul and is not to be touched. Not only did the nurse risk attracting the attention of dangerous spirits, but she also stroked the child in a taboo area.

Why did Mrs. Vo not come to visit her son in the hospital after she was discharged? She was probably practicing lying-in and was at home resting while her internal organs resumed their normal position in her body.

Nurses can best deal with Vietnamese mothers by following their lead. If the parents do not fuss over the child, nurses should not either. In any event, they should avoid touching the infant's head. And as long as a mother can feed and hold her baby properly, they should not be concerned about an apparent lack of interest. It is merely an illusion.

127   Nurses were similarly disturbed when an East Indian mother refused to hold her baby except to feed her. The nurses' concerns were quieted, however, when they later learned that the only care many Indian new mothers provide for their infants is to nurse them. A family member takes over its other care. In a variant of the lying-in period common throughout Asia and Latin America, the new mother is encouraged to rest in bed and eat a special diet including large amounts of milk, cooked butter, ghee (clarified butter), and high-protein foods.

Baby Naming

128   When the subject of baby naming came up in class, Leila, a Hindu nurse from India, shared her own experience. She said that when she and her husband had their first son, they wanted to name him in the traditional Hindu manner, which meant waiting until he was seven days old. Before choosing a name, they would have to consult an astrologer who would given them a list of auspicious letters, based upon the baby's time and date of birth. These letters would be given to her husband's sisters, who would then choose a name beginning with one of the letters on the list.

What they had not counted on was the response of the hospital. Despite the fact that Leila is a nurse, she did not realize the importance placed on filling out the birth forms. When they refused to fill in the baby's name, the nurse reported her to the head nurse. This resulted in visits from the hospital administrative nurse, the chaplain, and the social worker. They all seemed concerned about Leila's plans for the baby once they got home. When she asked the social worker why everyone seemed so disturbed, the social worker admitted that they were worried that she wasn't bonding properly with the baby—why else would she not have named him?

Leila and her husband were both shocked and embarrassed that anyone would think they did not want their child. She quickly explained the Hindu tradition to the social worker, who noted the information for the nursing staff. Leila also recommended that, in the future, if a patient refuses to fill out the child's name, they be asked *why* before any misundings result.

Leila was told to call the hospital as soon as they named the baby, but apparently, the hospital could not wait. On the morning of the seventh day, Leila received a call from the social worker, wanting to know the child's name so the forms could be completed.

When Leila asked her mother and grandmother why they were to wait until the seventh day to name the child, they told her that it is the day the stump of the umbilical cord falls off, and is thus the baby's first day of life. It is also the first time that the baby really opens his eyes and looks around. Although they did not mention it, it is probably related to high infant mortality rates.

This custom of delaying the name of the baby is found in many Asian cultures. Traditional Chinese will often give the baby an unattractive nickname at birth, such as "Little Doggie," or "Ugly Pig," to make the child seem less attractive to any spirits who might want to steal the infant.

Suk Luu, a Chinese man from Vietnam, shared that his mother attributes the fact that his daughter grew up to be healthy, talented, and intelligent to her "ugly" name; her "real" name was for use only on her birth certificate. As her grandmother explained, her ugly name insured that no devils paid attention to her; who would be jealous of an "ugly name girl"? In contrast, Luu's older brother was given a name that meant "intelligent" or "bright and clear." His mother pointed out that the devils were clearly jealous; his brother suffered serious illnesses for many years and died at the age of only thirty, as a military prisoner in South Vietnam.

129

Rejection

Occasionally parents will reject a newborn. Such was the case with a Middle Eastern couple after the wife, Salomi, gave birth to a baby girl. At the moment of delivery, while the doctor and nurses were oohing and aahing over the infant, her father turned and abruptly left the delivery room. Salomi herself would not hold or even look at her child. When a nurse approached the lobby where many of the woman's relatives had earlier been anxiously awaiting the birth, she found that they had all left. Later, Salomi held her child, but she refused to lavish any loving attention upon her.

130

The nurse who reported this incident could not understand why parents would respond so negatively to such a joyous event. A Middle Eastern acquaintance later told her the reason. Salomi and her husband had two daughters but no sons. Males are extremely important in Middle Eastern culture because they carry on the family name and all wealth is passed on through them. Many groups trace descent through the male line only, unlike our own system, which recognizes both the mother's and father's sides of the family. Even in groups that have adopted more Western patterns of inheritance, the traditional importance of the male may remain. For Salomi and her husband, a third daughter was a great disappointment.

There is little that the staff can do in such a situation, other than refer the parents to social services. Parents will rarely change ideas that have years of cultural tradition behind them. The important thing for nurses to do is to watch for signs of neglect.

Baby Care

131   In yet another case, a nurse attempted to explain baby care techniques to Middle Eastern parents. Since the new mother was not feeling well, the nurse began to explain everything to her husband. To the nurse's surprise, he refused to listen, stating that in his country men did not get involved in child care; it was a woman's job. Although economic and other factors may intervene, there is generally a very strict delineation of sex roles in the Middle East. Childrearing is a woman's responsibility. A man deals with his children later on in their lives. In such situations, it may be best to wait until a new mother is well enough to listen to instructions rather than try to explain things to her husband.

Breastfeeding

It is well known that the colostrum that fills a new mother's breasts before her milk comes in is rich in antibodies that fight infections to which newborns might be subject. Western doctors and nurses emphasize the importance of feeding infants colostrum. Many ethnic groups, however, refuse to do so.

132   Sofia Salgado, a Mexican American, gave birth to a son. The nurse wheeled the baby into Sofia's room and handed him to her to be nursed. Instead, Sofia pointed to her breasts and said, *"No leche, no leche"* (No milk, no milk). Pedro, her husband, explained to the nurse that Sofia would bottle-feed now and breastfeed when she returned home.

According to the nurse who related this example, most of the Mexican women who gave birth in a hospital near the Mexican border followed the same pattern—early bottle-feeding, later breastfeeding. Because colostrum is so important, this practice worries health care professionals.

Many Mexican women believe they have no milk until their breasts enlarge and they can actually see it. Some perceive colostrum as "bad milk" or "spoiled" and thus not good for a baby. Many do not realize that milk production is stimulated by nursing. Still others are very modest and are embarrassed to expose their breasts while nursing in the hospital.

The best way to deal with this situation is through education. Explain the importance of colostrum to the baby's health. If the mother's concern is to provide "real" milk for the baby, tell her that nursing on the colostrum will help it to come more quickly. The new mother should also be given privacy while nursing her infant.

133   Similar advice could be given to the Vietnamese mother who refused to breastfeed in the hospital, explaining that she would do so when she

returned home. The Vietnamese also believe that colostrum is dirty and often delay nursing until after their milk comes in.

Belly Buttons

American medical professionals fear germs. For this reason, they are almost obsessively concerned with cleanliness. A custom, practiced by Mexicans and other groups, designed to create an attractive belly button is thus likely to disturb them. A coin is applied to an infant's navel and the area is wrapped tightly with a cloth to keep the coin in place. Sometimes the job of keeping the navel flat is left entirely to the belly band. In any case, a protruding belly button is considered unsightly. Loving mothers will do what they can to ensure that their babies are attractive.

Health care professionals are concerned about the possibility of infection from a dirty cloth or coin. To respect their tradition and address health concerns, mothers who practice this custom should be taught the importance of using clean cloths and wiping the coin with alcohol before putting it on the baby's body. Most mothers are willing to make the minor adjustments necessary to ensure the health of their children.

Sterilization

A chapter on birth must also acknowledge efforts to prevent the event. Limiting the number of children is an extremely complicated issue in many cultures. Often, women and men take different positions on the issue, particularly in cultures where women have the primary responsibility for raising the children and men's major access to status and prestige is through the number of children they sire. Although a woman's status in such cultures may also derive from her role as a mother, women generally take the more practical stance.

Carmen, a twenty-four-year-old Mexican woman, was ready to deliver   134
her sixth child in six years. She begged her obstetrician to perform a tubal ligation after the delivery. Hospital policy, however, required Carmen's husband to sign a consent form for the procedure, and he would not allow it. Carmen was concerned that they would not be able to feed another child; she was not even sure they could feed this one. But her husband wanted as many children as Carmen could give him. She begged the physician to tie her tubes and not tell her husband.

He refused. The hospital had been sued by women who had been sterilized at their own request. The husband would learn later that his wife had had a tubal ligation. Rather than admit it had been done at her insistence and risk losing her husband, she would claim that she had not known what she was signing or had been coerced. For this reason, many hospitals now refuse to sterilize women without their husband's consent. (Interestingly, few, if any, hospitals, require the wife's consent for a vasectomy.)

135   A forty-five-year-old Mexican woman named Luna Ortiz was advised by her obstetrician that another pregnancy might prove fatal. Her eighth pregnancy (and third cesarean) had caused a thinning of her uterine wall. Rather than have her tubes tied while she was in the hospital, Mrs. Ortiz said she would have to discuss the matter with her husband. "He will decide what to do." Unlike Carmen, Mrs. Ortiz accepted the authority of the male to make all major decisions, including whether to have more children, regardless of how it affected her health.

Summary

Different cultures have different traditions regarding the process of birth. Some cultures dictate that a woman suffer the pains of labor in silence; others encourage her to express or even exaggerate her pain. The birth may be attended by the husband, mother, or mother-in-law. Some cultures have postpartum rituals that a new mother must observe which contradict the recommendations of Western medical science. Some bathe and exercise as soon as possible, while others are taught to lie in bed and avoid showering and physical activity. Some have customs which may appear to reflect a lack of bonding, but, in fact, do not. Although immediate breastfeeding is now encouraged by doctors, women in some cultures believe it is necessary to wait several days lest the "dirty" antibody-rich colostrum harm their child. Finally, many cultures do not share our advocacy of birth control, in part because children are a major source of self-esteem for those who would otherwise have no access to status.

Some of these differences affect the health of the mother or child but others do not. Health care professionals must learn to recognize the difference. Detailed explanations and compromise are necessary when good health is the issue; cultural relativism must be exercised when it is not.

For female "circumcision" (genital mutilation), see Chapter 7.
For pica, see Chapter 12.

Chapter 10
Death and Dying

In the past most people died at home, cared for by their families. Today however, people are dying more frequently in hospitals, cared for by professionals. Thanks to improved medical technology, people are also taking longer to die. This life transition is fraught with difficulties for most patients and their families. In addition, there are complications that can occur because cultural traditions vary so significantly in terms of a variety of issues, including whether or not to reveal the diagnosis to the patient, attitudes toward removing life support, expression of grief at the time of death, and beliefs and customs surrounding the moment of death.

Who Knows the Patient Is Dying?

Patty, a hospice nurse, was assigned to manage the home care of Maria, a monolingual Spanish-speaking Mexican woman with metastatic breast cancer. Although Maria was receiving both chemotherapy and radiation, the cancer was progressing rapidly. The family were close and loving, and were trying to manage without outside help. Maria was desperately fighting not to let her disease upset normal family routines.

After two weeks of managing the case, Patty sensed an underlying strain. She felt that, despite their outward appearance, the family were not coping as well as they pretended and were not receiving the support they needed. Maria was choosing to compromise her comfort in order to maintain her traditional role in the family as wife and mother; however, her exhaustion was making it increasingly difficult to do so. The rest of the family were having a hard time maintaining the illusion of normalcy, knowing that their lives were changing dramatically. In short, everyone was trying to protect everyone else but collapsing under the strain.

Patty called in Sandra, a bilingual / bicultural colleague. Maria was able

136

to talk more openly to Sandra than when family members were used as translators. She could also talk to her more openly about her needs for pain medication. To discuss this through her family would be to let down the pretense of normalcy. In cases such as these, the use of a third-party interpreter who is knowledgeable in both the language and culture is essential.

This case raises the issue of the degree of open discussion within the family regarding illness and death. In many cultures, it is common for a serious diagnosis, such as cancer, to be withheld from the patient and given only to the family. It may be seen as insensitive to tell a patient he or she is dying. It may be thought to create a sense of hopelessness and hasten the dying process. A Mexican American woman explained that the stress of knowing your condition will only cause you to get worse. moreover, the very devout may believe that only God knows when someone will die. For the health care staff, however, honoring the patient's culture may mean ignoring the American values of honesty and individualism as well as create potential legal complications regarding the patient's "right to know."

How can such a situation be handled? I was told of one hospital where the conflict between the patient's right to know and cultural traditions which forbid it is dealt with when the patient first enters the hospital, before being examined by the doctor. The patient is asked if there is a family member who should be given the pertinent information. If there is, the patient then signs a waiver to that effect.

137   Sometimes a family's refusal to allow the patient to be told he or she is dying can prevent that patient from receiving hospice care. Mrs. Hidalgo, an elderly Mexican woman, was dying of cancer. Her doctor spoke with her family about receiving hospice care. They liked the idea of having the hospice personnel provide her with medication to reduce her pain; however, there was a problem. In talking with the hospice organization, the family learned that before the hospice would accept Mrs. Hidalgo as a patient, she had to sign informed consent, acknowledging that she had a terminal condition and would die within six months. Since the family would not allow Mrs. Hidalgo to see the form (and prognosis), hospice care could not be given.

When dealing with dying patients, one should not be surprised to find the family insisting that the diagnosis be withheld from the patient. Sometimes, as in the case of Maria, it will the patient who tries to hide the seriousness of her condition from her family. Often, each may know the truth of the situation but try to hide it from the other. Sensitive health care providers will be open to discussing any concerns that the patient might raise when the family is not around, since the patient's impending death may not be a topic than can be openly discussed in the family's presence.

Removing Life Support

Religious and cultural prohibitions can also affect the removal of life support. A study done at a Los Angeles hospital found that members of a number of different ethnic groups were reluctant to remove life support, often due to the belief that it would interfere with God's will by taking away the possibility of a miracle. Other explanations included the belief that enduring suffering is a sign of strength and an opportunity to show courage and faith, and should not be taken from the patient. Still others were opposed to suggestions that they remove life support because they did not trust medical personnel, whom they felt were motivated by racism. Other, more unusual circumstances can contribute to a refusal to remove life support, as the next case illustrates.

Ngoc Ly, a twenty-five-year-old Vietnamese man, was hit by a car while riding his bicycle to work. Paramedics were able to resuscitate him, but the physician at the local trauma center determined that Ngoc was clinically brain dead. He placed him on life support until Ngoc's family could be notified.

An interpreter explained Ngoc's condition to his wife and parents. They nodded in understanding and quietly left the hospital. Normally, the staff neurosurgeon would then have pronounced Ngoc dead and removed him from the ventilator, but he was suddenly called to surgery.

Later that afternoon, Ngoc's family met with Dr. Isaacs, the physician they had spoken to earlier. Dr. Isaacs intended to tell them of the plan to pronounce Ngoc dead and discontinue the ventilator, but the Lys had other plans. They informed him that they had consulted a specialist who said this was not the right time for Ngoc to die. Dr. Isaacs was confused. What kind of specialist would make such a recommendation? An astrologer who had read Ngoc's lunar chart advised that his death be postponed until a more auspicious date.

The physician had never encountered a situation like the one now facing him. Fearing legal repercussions if he did not abide by the family's request, he agreed to keep Ngoc on life support until further notice. A little less than a week later, the Lys called to tell him that Ngoc could now die.

Most members of the staff were stunned by this incident. Ngoc's body was starting to decompose and smell. People looked up books on astrology and questioned Vietnamese co-workers. They learned that astrology is taken seriously by many Asians. When an important decision is to be

138

made, they will often consult a *bomoh* or *dukun* to interpret the astrological charts.

Although most people cannot predict or control the date of their death, simply knowing when someone has died can be helpful in terms of knowing what fate has in store for the deceased's descendants. If a person dies at the "proper" time, his or her children will be rewarded with good health and goodwill. If the time is inauspicious, the children will suffer financial losses, unhappy marriages, or similar negative fates. A *bomoh* can tell people what the future holds for them so they can be prepared.

The Ly family had an opportunity denied to most people. By delaying removal of Ngoc's life support, they could influence the fate of his descendants for generations. How could they not do everything possible to bring good luck to his children?

Expression of Grief

Individuals express grief in a number of different ways. Furthermore, culture may influence whether it is more appropriate to cry and wail without restraint or to present a stoic face to the world. The hospital culture tends to find the latter more admirable as well as easier to cope with, which can present problems when people from more expressive cultures die.

139   Mustafa Mourad, a Muslim Arab, was admitted to the oncology floor. A few weeks earlier, he had been diagnosed with extensive colon cancer. His family kept him at home until he went into a coma. Upon admittance, it was determined that he was a "no code," but little else had been discussed. There had been no time to develop rapport. Six to ten family members were at his bedside throughout the night.

At 2 A.M., the daughter ran to get the nurse—he had stopped breathing. When nurse confirmed that he had no pulse, several family members began to cry and wail loudly. The nurses tried to comfort them, but Mr. Mourad's son pulled them away. Soon the entire family joined in the wailing. The son asked the staff not to interfere, stating that the loud display was part of the grieving process. He added that it was necessary in order for his father's soul to be released.

The problem was that it was 2 A.M., and the wailing and crying were disturbing all the other, non-comatose patients, who were pushing their call buttons. They were angry, concerned, and frightened, and wanted to know what was going on. When the nurse asked the patient's son to have them please soften the noise, he became angry and accused her of being disrespectful.

The nurse had called Mr. Mourad's physician earlier to report the death. He instructed her to call the emergency room physician to pronounce the man dead. They were still waiting for him. Meanwhile, the nurse called the nursing supervisor. She also, unsuccessfully, tried to speak with the family about lowering the noise.

The doctor from the emergency room arrived nearly an hour later. When he requested they stop their wailing, they complied. He arranged to have the body moved to the chapel where they could continue their mourning without disturbing the other patients. The physician also instructed the nursing staff not to call the mortuary until told to do so by the family, which they did at 10 A.M. the next morning.

There are a number of cultural elements displayed in the Moustafa case. No plans had been made with the mortuary regarding the impending death because to do so would interfere with the will of Allah. The most disturbing element of the case for the staff was the loud crying. Wailing is an important cultural ritual. The nursing staff, unaware of this, was totally unprepared.

Another cultural aspect was the fact that the family ignored the requests of the nurses but complied with those of the physician. Arabs have a great deal of respect for authority—of physicians, not nurses. This is accentuated by the greater respect the culture has for men.

In this situation, the physician demonstrated an important understanding of cultural diversity and suggested a solution (moving to the chapel) which allowed the family to continue their ritual without compromising other patients. It is important to work within the culture rather than impose solutions from without.

The Moment of Death

The next three cases involve Gypsies. The first centered on a dying Gypsy queen, who was a patient in the intensive care unit. Several Gypsy women kept a vigil at Sylvia Romany's bedside, blocking the nurses' access. Finally, one of them explained that when the queen dies, her powerful soul will enter the body of the person physically closest to her. The women were all vying for that position. They certainly would not want her soul to enter the body of one of the nurses. The staff was frustrated, but there was little they could do for Mrs. Romany in any case. She died a few days later, and presumably her soul entered the body of the most determined Gypsy woman.

Philip Maturo, a Gypsy king in his late seventies, was brought to the hospital and diagnosed with pneumonia. The severity of his illness necessitated an oxygen tent. Clan members caused pandemonium; they

140

141

crowded into Mr. Maturo's room, blocked the doorways, and filled the cafeteria with their coffee cups and cigarette smoke. This behavior, however, was merely a nuisance. The greatest problem was that they insisted on keeping a candle on the shelf at the head of Mr. Maturo's bed. The nurses lived in fear that it would be lit while the oxygen was turned on and cause an explosion. Many animated discussions were held on this point, but the Gypsies were adamant. If their king died, the candle would be lit at the moment of death to guide his spirit to heaven. Fortunately, Mr. Maturo recovered and the hospital survived.

142   Another hospital witnessed a different Gypsy custom regarding death. When the end was imminent, the clan received the hospital's permission to move the king outside, bed and all. They felt this would help free the soul of their dying leader, now unencumbered by walls and ceilings.

143   Concern for the ability of the spirit to soar to freedom is common in many cultures. One nurse who worked at a hospital close to the Hoopa Indian reservation in Northern California told of how, when someone died, the nurses would open the windows to allow spirits to leave. The importance of this custom to the Native Americans made it difficult for her when she moved to a hospital where none of the windows opened.

The Number "Death"

144   A young Japanese woman named Kieko Ozawa was being wheeled into operating room 4 when she noticed the number over the door. She began to cry softly. The nurse became concerned and asked what was wrong. Kieko was embarrassed but explained that the Japanese character for the number 4 is pronounced the same as the character for the word "death." Already concerned about her health, Kieko was disturbed to be wheeled into a room labeled "death."

Although she said it was just a silly superstition, Kieko was unable to let go of her fear. The surgery went well despite the room number, but the patient suffered needless anxiety. Had the hospital personnel mentioned to Kieko that she was being scheduled for room 4, her feelings might have become known in time to reschedule her into a different operating room. Room number 3, for example, would have been appropriate because 3 in Japanese characters also means "life."

145   The same is true for the Chinese. In fact, one hospital situated in a largely Chinese neighborhood realized that they needed an in-service workshop on cultural diversity when a Chinese man on their Board of Directors became quite upset during his hospitalization. He had been put in room 444.

Whenever possible, avoid putting Chinese and Japanese patients in rooms with the number "4."

Post-Mortem

Most religions have rules regarding what can be done to the body after death. Although there will be variations according to how devout the family is, there are some practices which health care professionals can anticipate. Orthodox Jewish and Muslim patients may be opposed to organ donations and autopsies (unless required by law). According to Jewish belief, the body must be whole for resurrection if the messiah comes. For that reason, Jewish families may request that the deceased be buried with amputated limbs and bloody clothing (for example, if they died in an accident). Furthermore, many Jews believe that the body belongs to God, and we do not have the right to disfigure it without a good reason. Many Muslims feel that the body should be returned to Allah in the same shape in which it was given. Hmong families are also likely to refuse autopsies and organ donations because they believe that whatever is cut will be missing when they reincarnate.

Summary

Although this chapter has only touched on some of the issues that face caregivers when working with dying patients, it demonstrates the importance of culture in affecting people's attitudes and behavior in the face of death. At the same time, remember that culture does not explain everything; people's responses at this momentous life transition are often purely personal.

Chapter 11
Mental Health

The mental health profession is paying increasing attention to the effect of culture on individual psychology. Many graduate programs in clinical psychology now offer courses on treating clients from culturally diverse backgrounds. Knowledge of the range of what is considered "normal" is essential to effectively treating both private practice clients and hospital patients. Unfortunately, psychiatric diagnoses of foreign patients are often inaccurate, due to health care workers' ignorance of cultural patterns. This chapter will address some issues that relate to the mental health of patients.

Culturally "Normal" or "Mentally Ill"?

One definition of mental illness is behavior which deviates from the norm. Since each culture values different behavior in its members, what is considered normal in one culture may be perceived as deviant in another. In a culture which values emotional control, expressiveness can be seen as a sign of instability. In a culture which values independence, the desire to live with one's family after adolescence may be seen as something that needs to be worked on in therapy. When diagnosing patients, it is essential to distinguish mental illness from culturally supported behaviors and personality traits.

146   Esperlita, a Filipino nurse, began acting strangely. Her aunt and uncle had died in a fatal car crash on their way to Reno. A week after the funeral, Esperlita began to see visions of them. She would hear someone calling her name, smell the scent of her uncle's hair dressing, and feel a cold breeze on her face. The experience disturbed her so much that she began having trouble sleeping and was losing her appetite.

Esperlita shared her experience with Jackie, an Anglo American nurse, who strongly advised her to get psychiatric help. Jackie believed that the stress of her relatives' death was leading Esperlita to a nervous breakdown.

Esperlita related the same story to Araceli, a Filipino co-worker. Araceli had a completely different interpretation. She thought that Esperlita's dead relatives, having died in a foreign country and lacking the proper burial ritual, were having trouble making their journey into the next world. Or perhaps they simply wanted to say good-bye. Whatever the explanation, Araceli saw the experience as normal, not as a sign of impending psychosis.

Convinced of Araceli's interpretation, Esperlita and her family offered masses for her departed aunt and uncle over the next two weeks. They also lit candles on their graves each night. At the end of two weeks, the voices, visions, and scents disappeared. Esperlita could sleep undisturbed and her appetite returned.

What is interesting about this case is the difference in the interpretation of the same behavior by an Anglo American and by a Filipino. The former's culture does not allow for the existence of spirits; the latter's does. Seeing spirits is not interpreted as a sign of mental illness in cultures where people believe spirits exist.

Caught Between Cultures

With the increasing numbers of immigrants in this country comes the growing problem of children who are raised at home with one set of cultural values and are exposed to another set at school and with friends. This can create stress for first generation Americans.

Tammy Tang was born in China, but her family moved to the United States when she was in elementary school. Her parents were very traditional. Although she was now in college, she still lived at home. In fact, she attended the specific college she did because her parents would not let her enroll in any university that was too far from home for her to commute. She was not allowed to date and had a very early curfew. If she were living in China, these restrictions would not have been a problem; however, she was living in the United States. Most of her friends could date and stay out as late as they wanted. Many lived in the dorms or had their own apartments. Tammy felt a tremendous inner conflict. She respected and wanted to obey her parents; at the same time, she wanted the freedom enjoyed by most American college students.

She felt further trapped by her inability to discuss her feelings with anyone. It had been deeply ingrained in her that you never talk to outsiders about your problems; you discuss them only with your family. But her family *was* her problem. How could she talk to them? It would be completely disrespectful.

I know of Tammy's situation because she was a student in one of my classes. As part of a class requirement, she had to keep a journal. There were several entries in which she discussed her dilemma and the fact that she had often considered suicide as a solution. When I read these entries, I immediately asked Tammy to come see me. I told her that I understood her situation, and strongly advised her to seek help at the Student Counseling Center. Therapists who have worked with clients caught between cultures say that the most effective approach in dealing with such problems is a direct one: discuss the conflicts as resulting from cultural differences. It is not about being a "good" or "bad" person, but what is valued in different cultures

The wise health care provider will recognize the potential for such problems with their adolescent patients. The stress created by inter-generational, inter-cultural conflicts may be a complicating factor in presenting health problems. Social workers who are trained in cultural diversity may be needed. However, since people from many immigrant cultures have strong feelings against any kind of psychotherapy, because either "mental illness" is highly stigmatized or because personal problems should not be discussed with outsiders, any counseling sessions will have to be scheduled when the family are not around.

When Problems Go Undiagnosed or Untreated

148   A fifty-five-year-old Mexican American woman named Maria Ibañez was admitted to the coronary care unit with chest pain. She appeared withdrawn and was crying. When asked what was wrong, she shook her head and replied, "Nothing." She gave brief answers to Dr. Mandel, the physician who took her family history, but offered no additional information. Her crying continued even after her chest pain ceased, so Dr. Mandel asked why she was depressed. Still she did not answer.

Eventually Mrs. Ibañez's thirty-five-year-old daughter Cecilia arrived and explained that her mother had been in a state of emotional upset since her father had left home two weeks before. At this Mrs. Ibañez cried out, "No, no! You must not say anything. It's private." Cecilia quietly replied that she could not stand to see her mother suffer so and that she was frightened by her chest pains. Dr. Mandel then suggested that Mrs. Ibañez might want to talk with the staff psychiatrist. In response she exclaimed, "No! No other people should know about this!" Dr. Mandel drew Mrs. Ibañez closer to him, held her hand, and gently said, "Okay. But we need to talk about this." Cecilia, who was visibly disturbed, pleaded with her mother. "Please, Mama."

Why was Mrs. Ibañez so reluctant to discuss the problem that was most likely causing her chest pains? A Mexican nurse on staff later explained that Mexicans feel personal matters should be handled only within the family. They should not be discussed with strangers. Furthermore, a traditional Mexican woman's status is in large part derived from her role as a wife. If her husband leaves, she is nothing. Mrs. Ibañez's pride and embarrassment probably prevented her from talking about the situation. Her daughter, a second-generation Mexican American, was more Westernized and thus more open with outsiders about personal matters.

As it turned out, Mrs. Ibañez did not have a heart attack and was transferred to the post-coronary-care unit the next day. The nurse attending her case stopped by her room several times before she left. Although she still did not want to discuss her husband, she had stopped crying and was feeling somewhat better emotionally. What she needed most from the staff was nonintrusive warmth and support. In this case, the underlying emotional nature of the problem was discovered, due to the intervention of the more Westernized daughter and the sensitivity of the physician. However, had they not been involved, it is easy to see how the somatocization of Mrs. Ibañez's emotional condition could have easily masked the real problem.

It is important for health care providers to remember the strong connection between the mind and the body. People often somatocize their emotional stress. The potential for this is further increased when culture dictates a withholding of feelings. It may take a great deal of sensitivity and luck to get patients to discuss their feelings with health care providers. Whenever possible, try to involve culturally appropriate individuals, such as clergy members, traditional healers, or more acculturated family members.

Healer or Psychotic?

Juan Gutierrez, a fifteen-year-old Mexican American boy, was referred to the in-patient psychiatric unit of the hospital by his school psychologist. She noted that he had a history of seizures and was currently experiencing visual and auditory hallucinations as well as evidencing delusional thinking. Although they were very loving parents, the Gutierrezes were not in favor of the decision to hospitalize Juan and did not want him treated with medication. They did not share the hospital staff's view that he was mentally ill, despite the fact that he heard voices in his head, alternatively complimenting and criticizing him, and was constantly being distracted by things he alone could see. The staff also noted that Juan was experiencing delusions of grandeur, with his belief that he was born destined to be a *curandero* (traditional healer). In fact, his family reinforced this belief and interpreted what the staff saw as his "psychotic" symptoms as signs of his "calling."

Fortunately, the hospital staff in this situation acted in a culturally appropriate manner. Although they did not share Juan's interpretation of

149

his symptoms, and proceeded to put him on antipsychotic medication, they did follow the recommendation of a Mexican American therapist who suggested that a *curandero* meet with Juan and his family.

The meeting had a very positive effect on the mood and attitude of the entire Gutierrez family. Juan's symptoms showed gradual improvement, and he began to participate in the hospital's program of structured activities with his peers. Not long afterward he was able to be discharged home, on continued medication and with an appointment at his community mental health facility. In all liklihood, Juan also continued to see the *curandero*.

In the Realm of the Supernatural

150   Clara Sandoval, a seventy-one-year-old Mexican woman, was referred to a geriatric assessment program by a local psychiatrist. He had been treating her for severe depression using antipsychotic and antidepressant medications. They had not helped. In the past year she had lost forty pounds. She often lay awake at night, crying and screaming. Her doctor recommended in-patient hospitalization with electro-shock therapy, and sent her for assessment. Though uncomfortable with the doctor's recommendation, Mrs. Sandoval's family agreed to abide by the geriatric assessment program's recommendations.

When the geriatric assessment team arrived at Mrs. Sandoval's home, they found her in a darkened room filled with religious icons. She was wearing a six-inch crucifix around her neck. During her two-hour interview, Mrs. Sandoval wrapped her rosary around her hand and began to beat her chest. She frequently referred to the "evil ones" who were stealing her soul and the "voices" that haunted her in the night. Her affect during the interview ranged from flat and unresponsive to near hysteria. Mrs. Sandoval's family added that, although she had been a devout Catholic, she refused to go to mass during the past year and would not accept any visits from the local clergy.

When they spoke with the parish priest, he told the assessment team that it was not uncommon for elderly Hispanic women to fear possession and punishment for past sins. He supplied them with the name of an exorcist who had successfully treated some of these cases. The exorcist visited Mrs. Sandoval on three occasions. Although it is not known what he did during those visits, when the geriatric assessment team visited Mrs. Sandoval a month later, they found her remarkably improved. Her antidepressant medication appeared to be working, and she had gained ten pounds.

Exactly what happened in this case is unclear. What is known is that an obviously religious woman had been suffering from depression, was hearing voices, and feared that her soul was being taken by "evil ones." Medication was ineffective in treating her condition. After three visits from an exorcist, she was on the road to recovery. The important point is that treatment within the framework of Mrs. Sandoval's belief system was effective in a way that traditional psychiatric treatment was not.

A similar situation occurred with Carlos Gonzales, a twenty-two-year-old Mexican American inmate of the county jail. He was referred to medical services with symptoms of a heart attack. When the doctor examined him, he discovered no cardiac abnormalities. Carlos was then sent to the mental health section, where he appeared to be in a state of acute fear. He clutched his left side, and his garbled Spanish was incoherent. From his appearance and vital signs, alcohol withdrawal was suspected. He was sent back to the medical service.

151

Shortly thereafter, Carlos was returned to the mental health service. He lay on the floor, conscious but shaking violently, a look of terror covering his face. He claimed to be dying and begged Regina, the nurse, to inform his mother. Asking Carlos if he believed in God and getting an affirmative answer, Regina reached for a Bible. She quickly tore out a picture of Jesus and held it over his heart. Slowly he calmed down. When asked if he wanted a cigarette, Carlos surprised everyone by getting up and following Regina to her office.

Still clutching Jesus' picture to his chest, Carlos explained that he had been cursed by a former lover in Mexico. When he ended the relationship, she consulted a *bruja* (witch) who put a spell on him that would cause him to die of a heart attack. Regina called Carlos's home and spoke with his sister, who confirmed the story.

As the night wore on, Carlos gradually stopped shaking but remained fearful. Regina finally convinced him that his belief in God, coupled with the prayers of his family, would counteract the curse. By morning, he was fairly calm, perhaps because he was still alive.

Interpreting the incident from an etic perspective, one might suggest that Carlos experienced heartburn that evening. Mindful of the curse, he thought his symptoms signaled a heart attack. His Catholicism may have also contributed to his guilt, punishing his "love" affair with a "heart" attack. From an emic perspective, the *bruja* worked a powerful spell.

Anthropological Perspectives on the Supernatural

From an anthropological perspective, it is somewhat difficult to discuss cases involving the supernatural. If one acknowledges the reality of the supernatural, one is not being scientific; if one does not, one is being ethnocentric. If in fact such things as spirits and witchcraft exist, the responses of Carlos and Mrs. Ibañez are perfectly normal, and do not belong in a chapter on "Mental Health," except in terms of how their behavior is interpreted by the dominant American culture.

The symptoms Juan experienced are certainly consistent with that of receiving a spiritual "calling." In fact, it is common for shamans to experience psychotic episodes before they begin shamanizing. It is through these episodes that they learn to control their entrance into and out of altered states of consciousness which psychiatrists refer to as "psychotic." Often the problem with psychotics is that their perceptions do not "match" those of the rest of us, they therefore cannot function in our society. It has been argued that by acknowledging "hallucinations" and "delusions" as real—as evidence of communication with the spirit world—nonwestern societies provide a place for psychotics to function. That view, however, is rather ethnocentric. If we are to be culturally relativistic, we should not dismiss entirely the possibility that there is a spirit world and that some people have the ability to connect with it.

Because we do not recognize shamanic healers, witchcraft, or "evil ones" in our own culture, we have no framework for understanding the experiences of Clara Sandoval, Carlos Gonzales, or Juan Gutierrez beyond that of psychosis. It is unknown what the visiting *curandero* said or did with the Gutierrez family. However, at the very least, it is clear that the fact that the acknowledgment by hospital staff of the family's belief system made them much more cooperative and comfortable. From the medical perspective, it was the medications that helped Juan, but his attitude after seeing the *curandero* certainly may have contributed to a faster and smoother recovery, as well as to his willingness to participate in the medical treatment plan.

The lesson to be learned from all these cases is that, whatever one's personal world view, it is far more effective to treat patients in the context of their belief system rather than just one's own.

Summary

The crux of the mental health issue rests with what is considered normal. Because this varies cross-culturally, behaviors which are perceived as normal in one culture are deemed abnormal in another. This becomes a problem in the United States because of the vast numbers of people from diverse cultures living here. While there are some individuals who would be considered mentally ill in *any* culture, there are many who are labelled mentally ill because their beliefs or behavior are not consistent with cultural norms. For example, a person who has visions of the dead may be perceived as abnormal, normal, or even special, depending on the beliefs of the culture. Health care providers who understand the world view of their patients will generally have much more success in treating them.

Health care workers also need to be sensitive to the fact that mental illness is highly stigmatized in many cultures; patients with emotional problems may be reluctant to discuss them with strangers. This can be a particular problem for the children of immigrants, who may feel unable to discuss the stress they experience resulting from the conflict between American culture and that of their parents. In all cases, what is called for is greater awareness and sensitivity on the part of the health care provider.

Chapter 12
Folk Medicine—Practices and Perspectives

One source of misunderstanding in the hospital stems from the practice of various folk treatments. Some can result in misdiagnosis; others simply contradict scientific medicine. Misunderstandings can also arise from patients' beliefs about the proper use of prescribed medications. Such beliefs and practices are the focus of the first part of this chapter.

A second topic concerns the concept of body image. The ideal image varies considerably from culture to culture and may affect patients' attitudes toward specific treatments.

Coin Rubbing

152   A thirty-eight-year-old Cambodian male was brought into the hospital, semicomatose, with rows of red marks on his body. He was suffering from severe headache, nausea, vomiting, and lethargy. Once he was hospitalized, one of his relatives began to rub the marks on his skin with something that looked like oil.

153   The adult children of a Vietnamese woman rushed their mother to the hospital. The emergency room personnel discovered dark red welts running up her arms, shoulders, and chest, yet her only presenting complaint was dizziness. When questioned, her son explained that he had rubbed her body with a quarter.

154   A nurse became concerned when she found an elderly Chinese patient rubbing himself with a quarter; she thought he was trying to hurt himself. When she took the coin away from him, he became very upset, grabbed it back from her, and continued to rub his arms and legs, leaving dark red scratches.

In each case, the nurses responded with a combination of disbelief, disgust, curiosity, ridicule, intolerance, and finally attempts to understand. In each case, the explanation was the same. The patients were practicing a traditional Asian form of healing known as coin rubbing.

There are several variations, including heating the coin or putting oil on it, but they all involve vigorously rubbing the body with a coin. This produces red welts on the affected area, which can distract health professionals from the real problem or be mistaken for child abuse.

Underlying this practice is the belief that the illness in the body needs to be drawn out. Rubbing the body with a coin produces a raised red area, giving the appearance that the illness has been brought to the surface of the skin. It is believed that red marks will appear only on people who are ill, which is seen as further support for the effectiveness of the technique. Many Asian Americans claim that they still practice coin rubbing because it brings relief from colds and other ailments.

Lack of knowledge of this widespread practice can have disastrous results. A Korean man named Sung Kim was brought into the emergency room, unconscious. His chest was covered with red welts. The family did not speak English, and there was no interpreter available. The staff assumed that Mr. Kim's lack of consciousness was related to the red welts, that both were symptoms of the same condition. They were not. Unfortunately, by the time they discovered what Mr. Kim was suffering from, it was too late to help him. Had they known to ignore the welts, they might have saved his life.

A Vietnamese girl named Kathy Dinh was in her first year at an American elementary school. She was not feeling very well one morning so her mother rubbed the back of her neck with a coin. She then felt well enough to attend school. Later in the day, however, she began to feel worse and went to see the school nurse. When the nurse discovered the welts on Kathy's neck, she immediately assumed she was seeing a case of child abuse and conscientiously reported the Dinhs to the authorities. The situation was finally straightened out, but it created a great deal of needless embarrassment for Kathy's family.

It is not that Asians never abuse their children, but rubbing them with coins is not the way they do it, any more than Americans abuse their children by having thin pieces of metal wrapped around their teeth and tightened until their teeth move out of place. Braces are often applied for primarily aesthetic reasons. Coin rubbing, at least, is an attempt to heal. Apparently, it often works; only the failures show up in the medical system.

It is important that health care professionals become familiar with the practice, lest they become distracted from the real problem or mistakenly make accusations of child abuse. When such welts are observed, if the patient and family do not speak English, it would be a good idea to pull out a coin and mime rubbing the body with it. That, along with a questioning look, would probably convey the message. If the patient or family nods in agreement, the marks should be ignored. If it is necessary to write a report on the marks, a note should be made indicating that they may be the result of a traditional healing practice.

Cupping

157   Another healing method that produces similarly misleading results is cupping. John Bagdasarian, a forty-six-year-old Armenian, was brought into the critical care unit with a diagnosis of acute myocardial infarction (heart attack). While doing a physical assessment, the nurse found round red marks all over his upper back which looked like burns. The staff speculated about the source of the marks. Theories ranged from birthmarks to some form of torture or sadism. An Armenian physician finally cleared up the mystery. The marks were a result of cupping.

The patient's family had tried to cure him of his chest pains by heating a glass and placing it on his body. The vacuum created under the glass caused the skin to rise and left the red marks. What did the Bagdasarians hope to accomplish with this procedure? Possibly they believed that John's pain was caused by cold air entering his chest. Applying a hot glass on the back is thought to equalize the imbalance in the body. Another possibility is that it was done to chase out the evil spirit that was causing the pain. In any case, when cupping did not stop the chest pains, his family brought him to the hospital.

Cupping is said to be particularly successful for treating sore muscles and is frequently practiced for that purpose in many parts of the world, including Asia, Latin America, and parts of Europe, and is taught in acupuncture colleges in the United States. As with coin rubbing, however, cupping can easily be misinterpreted by health care professionals who are not aware of the practice.

Fevers

Current medical wisdom has it that the most effective way to reduce fever is to cool the body. This is done by removing regular blankets and placing an "ice blanket" under the patient. In contrast, many cultures believe that the best way to treat a high temperature is to sweat it out. These conflicting theories are the source of another common cultural conflict in the hospital.

158   Hiroshi Tomita, a Japanese businessman on a trip to the United States, was admitted to the hospital with a 102-degree fever of unknown origin. According to standard procedure, his nurse, Jean, removed the blankets from the bed, leaving only a sheet to cover him. She explained that it was to keep his temperature from going up. She gave him a glass of cold

apple juice, but he only took two sips. At 9 P.M., the doctor examined Mr. Tomita and prescribed a mild analgesic every four hours for temperatures greater than 101 degrees and a cooling blanket for temperatures greater than 102 degrees. When his temperature rose to 103 degrees at 10 P.M., Jean ordered a cooling blanket, per the doctor's instructions. At this point, Mr. Tomita asked for his blankets, but Jean refused, once more explaining why. She put the ice blanket under him and left the room. In a few minutes, Mr. Tomita complained that the ice blanket was too cold and asked for his regular blankets. For the third time, Jean patiently explained the treatment. He did not say anything; he simply curled up under his sheet. When Jean returned a half hour later to check on him, he was sitting up in the chair with all the blankets wrapped around him, covered with goose bumps and shivering. By midnight, his temperature was up to 105 degrees. Jean gave him his second dosage of acetaminophen. Mr. Tomita continued to ask for his blankets and to get out of bed. Jean was at the point of putting restraints on him to keep him in bed.

She asked him why he did not want to stay in bed. He explained that in Japan, people with fevers were covered with warm blankets and given plenty of hot drinks. Cold juice was particularly inappropriate. This approach, found throughout Asia, is probably based on the Chinese notion of hot and cold balance, or yin and yang. Mr. Tomita was experiencing chills, which logically should be treated with heat, not cold. Furthermore, it is believed that fevers must be sweated out, again necessitating measures that produce greater warmth.

Reflecting on his comment, Jean asked herself what she did when suffering from a temperature and chills. She realized that she did exactly what her patient wanted—she piled lots of blankets on herself, turned up the electric blanket to the maximum temperature, and drank hot liquids!

She then called a team conference. Most of her colleagues admitted to similar behavior, but no one wanted to take responsibility for going against medical orders. Realizing that she could no longer treat Mr. Tomita against his beliefs and wishes, Jean decided to call the admitting doctor. It was now 1 A.M. The physician was angry at being awakened. He impatiently listened to her story, was silent for a moment, and then agreed to a change in orders: discontinue the cooling blanket, administer analgesic tablets every three hours if the patient's temperature rose above 101 degrees, and keep the patient as comfortable as possible.

Mr. Tomita was extremely happy and grateful for the change in orders. His temperature came down after about three hours and eventually he removed the blankets on his own.

159   A similar case involved Rosa Torres, a twenty-nine-year-old Hispanic woman with a surgical infection. Rosa's temperature was 104 degrees. She had piled six blankets on top of herself, curled up into a ball, and lay there moaning loudly. When Rebecca, her nurse, discovered the mound of blankets, she attempted to remove them. Rosa vehemently refused. "No, I will get cold." Rebecca explained that the blankets were keeping her body temperature too high; she needed to remove them to reduce the fever. The explanation did nothing to change Rosa's mind, but Rebecca was determined and gently pulled off all but one blanket.

Shortly thereafter, Rebecca tried to take Rosa's temperature rectally, per the doctor's orders. Again, Rosa refused. She did not want her underwear removed and certainly did not want anyone to insert a rectal thermometer. Each of Rebecca's attempts to do so were met with screams. Rebecca tried to explain the importance of the greater accuracy of the rectal temperature, but Rosa did not care. Rebecca finally gave up, respecting Rosa's right to refuse. Another nurse on the unit, however, was not about to give in to the patient's desires and insisted that she remove her underwear. She managed to insert the thermometer despite Rosa's cries and tears.

Although Rebecca did not understand the reason for Rosa's behavior at the time, she later learned from several Hispanic friends that it is believed that one of the greatest dangers during a fever is letting in cold air. Removing all the covers thus put the patient at risk. Second, the illness is seen as a kind of poison. Keeping the blankets on causes the body to sweat out the poison; thus, the fever goes down and the illness disappears. Rosa's refusal to remove her underwear and have her temperature taken rectally was probably due to the modesty typically found among Hispanic women, along with the discomfort and sense of indignity involved.

Unlike the previous example, in which the nurse finally did respect the patient's wishes, in this case, Western medicine won out. Rosa was labeled a difficult patient because of her desire to adhere to her traditional beliefs regarding treatment of disease. Rebecca later suggested that the doctor could have been called to change the order from a rectal to an oral temperature. She still felt it was necessary to remove the blankets but thought that if she had understood Rosa's reasons, she might have been more empathetic.

160   In another case, a Mexican American mother refused to use cooling measures in caring for her febrile infant, despite medical instructions to do so. Mrs. Lopez had called the hospital because her infant's temperature was very high. She was told to give the baby a mild analgesic and a cool bath and then to bring her in. Mrs. Lopez ignored both cooling instructions and, to the consternation of the medical staff, brought the

child wrapped in several layers of blankets, outer garments, undershirt, and several pairs of socks. When asked why she did not follow the instructions given her, she replied, "He must sweat the fever out. Besides, he could get pneumonia from the night air and die."

Nurses who work in hospitals serving a large Hispanic population say that they see this behavior quite frequently. In fact, the sight of a family walking up to the registration window with a bundle of blankets in their arms usually prompts the nurses to prediagnose the child as having a fever and admit it right away. Immediate action is necessary to make sure the baby does not have a seizure while the family is registering.

Parents are generally willing to listen to the nurses' explanations on how to treat fevers in infants. The problem is often with their own parents. One young woman explained that she knew she should not wrap her baby so heavily, but her mother-in-law "made her do it." She had attended some parenting classes and knew the proper procedure but felt it was too difficult to fight the whole family. Health education is the only way to deal with such situations, but it will not be easy to overcome years of tradition.

Another example occurred with a Black woman and her tiny grandson. The child was brought into the hospital by his mother, Mary, and grandmother, Adele Wilson. The nurse explained that she would put the naked infant in a cool mist tent and bathe him in cold water to reduce his temperature. Mary was quiet, calm, and cooperative. She indicated her concern by asking several questions about her son's condition.

Adele Wilson, however, did not appear to be listening. She got up from her chair, looked into the tent, and said, "You forgot to give him a blanket. That thing is real cold inside." The nurse again explained that she was keeping him cool because of his high temperature. Mary tried to calm her mother-in-law, seeing that she was becoming hostile. "Mama, it's okay." Mrs. Wilson responded, "What you talkin' 'bout? They got you believing in this foolishness too. I'm gonna put his blanket on him 'cause he is cold. I raised all my nine children and I never put one in no ice box. You know you need to wrap him so he can sweat the fever out. Hot chamomile tea would bring that fever down."

Most of the nurses dealt with the grandmother by avoiding her. They could not talk to her without arguing. How might they have handled the situation? They might have begun by asking her how she would have treated the child. They could have acknowledged her approach, which comes from years of use of natural remedies within the Black culture. They might also have incorporated her recommendation of chamomile tea. Mrs. Wilson's hostility may have been a reaction to what she perceived as racism on the part of the white nurses. A bit more respect on the part of the nurses might have helped.

Pica

162   Ruth Clay, a twenty-eight-year-old paraplegic Black female with two children, craved Argo laundry starch while she was hospitalized following an
auto accident. Since she had few visitors, she asked the staff to bring her
the starch. The staff, who thought this craving was "crazy," told her they
did not have any. Furthermore, her renal disease dictated a limited diet.

Ruth became very depressed during her long hospitalization. Finally,
a young Black female physician was assigned to her case. Recognizing
Ruth's craving as a cultural practice, she recommended that the grateful
patient be allowed a small amount.

Eating laundry starch is a common form of pica—a craving for nonfood substances—among Black women, who often consume it during
pregnancy. Some think it helps "build up the blood." Others say it keeps
the baby's skin "clean." (It has a smooth, clean feel.) Still others believe
it helps settle the stomach. (The consistency is reminiscent of chalky ant-
acids.) This practice is a carryover from the slave tradition of eating dirt.
The clay dirt in the South is rich in iron, and the craving is generally
thought to be due to anemia or iron deficiency. (In truth, the ferric form
of iron [red, rust] is virtually unabsorbable and of no nutritional use.
The absorbable form is the ferrous ion. Therefore, eating soil would be
of no nutritional value, even in iron deficiency anemia.) When Blacks
moved out of the South, Argo starch (probably the major brand of laundry starch at the time) was substituted.

Although the circumstances under which the patient craved laundry
starch were unusual, her choice of that particular nonfood item was not.
In her mind, it may have been associated with a happier time—pregnancy—and thus brought her some consolation during this very difficult
time. Psychologically, this is similar to the common practice of eating
"comfort foods" when we are depressed. These are the special foods that
our mothers made us eat when we were children, foods we associate with
love and warmth.

Folk Healers

163   Another potential area for misunderstanding or confusion involves the
use of folk healers. A sixty-year-old Black woman named Pearl Smith was
admitted to the critical care unit with severe diarrhea and dehydration. All
tests and exploratory surgery were negative. In desperation, the family
called in a voodoo doctor. The staff reacted with disbelief, especially
since the patient was educated and upper middle class. How could they
seriously consult a "witch doctor?"

Since orthodox medicine had ruled out all medical causes, the only other possibility was a magical cause. Perhaps someone had put a hex on Mrs. Smith. Belief in voodoo often persists in Black culture, despite education and social class—just as do superstitious beliefs in Anglo culture. Like most ethnic groups, Blacks often use multiple health care systems simultaneously. One student shared that his Mexican grandmother will see a doctor when ill and go to the hospital if necessary, but will also say the appropriate prayers and light candles to help her get well. If she does not recover, she generally attributes it to not lighting enough candles or reciting a sufficient number of prayers.

To return to the case of Mrs. Smith, did voodoo succeed where orthodox medicine failed? In this case, both systems were unsuccessful. Mrs. Smith continued to waste away and died several months after the onset of her illness.

The story of an eighty-three-year-old Cherokee Indian woman named Mary Cloud has a happier ending. Her grandson Joe brought her into the hospital emergency room after she had passed out at home. Lab tests and x-rays indicated that she had a bowel obstruction. After consulting with Joe, the attending physician called in a surgeon to remove it. Joe was willing to sign consent for the surgery, but it would not be legal; the patient had to sign for herself. Mrs. Cloud, however, refused; she wanted to see the medicine man on the reservation. Unfortunately, it was an hour and a half drive each way, and she was too ill to be moved. Finally, the social worker suggested that the medicine man be brought to the hospital.

Joe left and drove to the reservation. About three hours later he returned, accompanied by a man in full traditional dress complete with feather headdress, rattles, and bells. He entered Mrs. Cloud's room and for forty-five minutes conducted a healing ceremony. Outside the closed door, the stunned and amused staff could hear bells, rattles, chanting, and singing.

At the conclusion of the ceremony, the medicine man informed the doctor that Mrs. Cloud would now sign the consent form. She did and was immediately taken to surgery. Her recovery was uneventful and without complications.

What was responsible for her recovery? The hospital staff were sure it was the skill of the surgeon; Mrs. Cloud was convinced it was a result of the power of the medicine man. In any case, without the medicine man she would not have agreed to the surgery or, if she had, her attitude might have been so poor as to interfere with recovery. This is a perfect example of how traditional healers and physicians can successfully work together in the care of patients.

164

how is this different from a priest?

Medications: Improper Use

165   A common source of cross-cultural misunderstandings involves the use
of Western medications, which often differs from the application of traditional remedies. It is essential that complete explanations be given to
patients regarding how to use medication. Florence, a Black nurse, was
doing home care for a thirty-year-old Mexican female named Lena Menendez who had recently had a cesarean section. Mrs. Menendez spoke
little English. Her mother, Gloria Flores, was staying with her to help with
the baby. During her first visit, she wanted to make an assessment evaluation and change the dressing on the incision site.

When Mrs. Menendez removed her underpants, the first thing Florence noticed was the absence of a pad or gauze covering the gauze inside
the wound. When she looked more closely, she discovered a bloody white
cheesy substance on the gauze and in the corners and edges of the
wound. Florence had no idea what it was. In her mind, she considered
the possibilities: semen? intestines? When she removed the old dressing,
she was relieved to find that it was not her intestines. She could find no
evidence of infection, and after cleaning the wound, decided it was just
a dirty wound.

When Florence returned the next day, she noted more of the white,
bloody, cheesy substance. This time, she asked Mrs. Menendez what it
was. Her mother answered for her, replying, "Her medication, the one
with the powder in it. The nurse said it was for infections." Florence was
astounded. She explained that the medication was to be taken by mouth.
Mrs. Flores said, "No, in my culture, we mix the powder and put it where
the infection is. In order for the wound to heal, the powder goes in
there." Florence then spent several minutes explaining to Mrs. Flores
and her daughter the difference between American medicine and traditional Mexican medicine. It was unfortunate that the nurse who had
given her the medication had neglected to explain how it is used. Moreover, Florence should have asked about it on the first visit.

Do not assume that a patient will understand how to take the medication prescribed. Medicines are used in different ways in different
countries, and confusion can result. Alternately, people simply may be
unfamiliar with the administration of medicinal products, as evidenced
in the next two cases.

166   One nurse related the case of an angry Mexican woman who became
pregnant even though she faithfully took her birth control pill every day.
Questioning revealed that the woman had inserted the pills into her vagina. Her action may have seemed logical to her; unfortunately, it was
not effective.

167   Another Mexican woman became pregnant while using contraceptive

foam. Although the failure rate with foam is much higher than with birth control pills, that was not the cause of her pregnancy. No one had explained to her how to use the foam. Since the directions on the can were in English, which she did not understand, she and her husband did what made sense to them— they applied the foam to his penis before he inserted it into her vagina. Again, when giving information on the use of any kind of medication, it is extremely important to give clear and complete instructions on its use.

Medications: Noncompliance

Health care practitioners are often frustrated when patients do not follow through on their prescriptions. Sometimes, this apparent noncompliance can result from cultural factors. Recall the case described earlier involving Mrs. Nyguen, the sixty-five-year-old Vietnamese refugee. In addition to her lung problems, she was also dehydrated and malnourished. She ate little and did not comply with the dietitian's recommended liquid supplement.

168

While interviewing the patient regarding her condition and health care practices, the nurse learned that she was drinking rice water as a remedy for her gastrointestinal tract. Although her physician had given her a prescription for medication, Mrs. Nyguen was not familiar with the procedure of having a prescription filled, and had put the prescription with the rest of the indecipherable papers they had received at discharge.

There is an important lesson in this case. Realize that recent immigrants may not be familiar with the system of having prescriptions filled, since they may have always been given medications directly by the doctor. Be sure to explain the procedure.

In another example of "noncompliance," an Anglo American nurse named John was caring for an older African American patient named Robert Williams. Mr. Williams had been admitted for congestive heart failure. Apparently he had not been taking several of the medications his doctor had prescribed. When John asked why, he explained that he only took his "breathing pill" (digoxin) when he became short of breath. He did not see why he had to take it every day, even when he had no symptoms. It is important that health care providers explain the reason for taking each medication, particularly those which only have a preventive function.

169

Scars

Most Americans are concerned with their appearance. Surgeons, therefore, try to leave as small a scar as possible. This effort had a negative

170

effect with a forty-one-year-old Nigerian patient named Osito Seisay, who was introduced in Chapter 3. He had come to the United States to have his brother operate on his knee, which was injured when a bull charged him.

His nurse was concerned when he did not request pain medication following surgery. She learned the reason when his sister-in-law came to visit and spoke to Mr. Seisay in his native language. He was enduring the pain as an offering to Allah.

The next cultural incident occurred when Mr. Seisay's brother, the surgeon, came to remove the bandages. He was very proud of his work and pointed out how small the surgical scar was. Mr. Seisay, however, did not share his brother's happiness. He was disappointed over the small size of the scar. He felt that without a large scar to mark the surgery, the other members of his tribe would not believe he had suffered very much. What kind of offering to Allah would that be?

His brother had obviously shed most of the old tribal ways. He could not believe Osito still held these beliefs and tried in vain to convince him otherwise. At this point, nothing could be done. One would think that Mr. Seisay's brother, being aware of tribal customs, would have anticipated Osito's response. He did not. He was too Westernized. Surgeons, however, should be aware that all patients do not share the same ideal body image and should discuss such things in advance.

Fat

171   Mention of ideal body image brings up the subject of fat. American culture values thinness and views obesity as a disease. Many cultures, however, see thinness as a problem and plumpness as the ideal. Jane, a nurse, was about fifty pounds overweight. She was embarrassed about her size and eventually managed to lose most of the excess weight. She related an incident that occurred when she was at her heaviest.

Her Panamanian boyfriend, Mario, brought her home to meet his family. When they saw her, they were delighted that she was so fat. They told her this several times during the evening. Jane was totally humiliated by their remarks. She was already nervous about meeting Mario's family, and now they were insulting her. Yet they seemed so friendly.

Near the end of the evening, Mario, sensing her discomfort, took her aside and explained. In his culture, fat is seen as healthy. A fat woman can have lots of babies. All his other girlfriends had been far too thin to suit his family. At last, he was going out with a "real woman." They had not been insulting her by calling her fat; they were bestowing a great compliment. His explanation made Jane feel a little better, though their repeated comments about her size continued to disturb her.

Although this incident did not take place in the hospital, it illustrates a problem that could arise there. Most Latin Americans and Eastern Europeans, among others, share Mario's family's view of body size. Advice that a patient lose weight might not be followed because it would create a negative body image. Imagine a slim American woman being told she should gain twenty-five pounds for the sake of her health. How willing would she be to trade her "attractive" figure for one that she sees as too fat? Health care professionals should be aware of possible resistance and be prepared to deal with it.

Bathroom Behavior

The last incident to be discussed in this chapter does not fit neatly into any of the categories covered. It involves elimination. The patient, Hyun Kim, a seventy-four-year-old Korean man, had come to the United States to visit his family. While here, he became ill and had to be hospitalized for renal and respiratory failure. He was put on strict bed rest because exertion would be dangerous. Conflict arose because several times a day, his family got him out of bed to squat over the bedpan on the floor. Kate, his nurse, tried to explain that the bedpan was to be used in bed, but they did not speak much English and became very upset. Kate was mystified over Mr. Kim's behavior.

A Filipino co-worker later explained. In most Asian countries, traditional toilets are holes in the ground. To eliminate from the bowels, one squats over the hole. There is no other way to do it. Until recently, most people did not have toilets inside their homes; they were located outside. Even today, the toilet is kept separate from the tub or shower. One is for cleansing, the other for waste. Elimination is considered unclean and certainly should not be done in bed. Mr. Kim's family was simply trying to maintain standards of cleanliness and decency. Mr. Kim was using the bedpan in the only way he knew how.

Once Kate understood his behavior, she drew the curtains around him for privacy. She then spoke to the physician and had him rewrite the orders from strict bedrest to bathroom privileges as needed with assistance. Mr. Kim and his family were much happier and more cooperative as a result. Kate also felt better because she was no longer frustrated over her lack of control.

More than once I have had the experience of going into a public restroom, checking the floor of the stalls for an empty one and, having found it, opened the door to find an Asian woman with her feet on the seat, squatting over the toilet. It is biomechanically easier to move the bowels in this position and is common in many parts of the world where Western plumbing is not found—and, occasionally, where it is. I was in a

172

museum in southern France several years ago. I went to use the restroom but could not find the toilet. Finally, someone pointed out a hole in the ground. There were depressions on either side in the shape of foot-prints. I had to overcome a great deal of ethnocentrism before I was able to use it. The experience did, however, help me to be more understanding when I open a stall door to discover a woman with her feet on the toilet seat.

Summary

Most medical personnel believe that Western scientific medicine is superior to all other medical systems. In some cases, this may be true. It is important to remember, however, that medical practitioners in other cultures have been treating patients with some success for centuries. Several modern drugs, including quinine, were discovered in native "medicine kits." Furthermore, scientific medicine has been notably unsuccessful in curing many ailments, including the common cold.

Even in cases where Western scientific medicine is superior, if the patient believes it is insufficient for treating the problem, it probably will be. The mind has a powerful effect on the body and can influence both illness and health. To treat patients successfully, it is extremely important to take their beliefs into account, whether they be about the causes of disease, how it should be treated, what behavior is appropriate, or how the body is viewed.

Ideally, medical professionals everywhere will recognize the value of what other systems have to offer. They can then take the best of each and reach the ultimate goal of providing effective health care for all.

For more on medications, see Chapter 3.
For more on folk healers, see Chapter 11.

Chapter 13
Conclusion

The examples in this book are by no means exhaustive. They represent a small sampling of the problems that can occur between members of different ethnic groups. Many of the basic principles that are illustrated by the examples can help in interpreting other conflicts or, ideally, preventing further misunderstandings. The works listed in the bibliography should help the interested reader research other aspects of cultural differences.

One of the issues that often arises in class discussions is that of ethics. Why should the Western health care system adapt to the needs of other cultural groups? We hear complaints such as, "Why don't they adapt to our ways?" "Why don't they learn to speak English? My grandparents did." Certainly, hospitals in most other countries are not nearly so accommodating to patients of other cultures.

One response is to say, yes, they should adapt to our culture and learn our language. That is not, however, the most compassionate or practical response. It is the goal of the medical profession to provide optimal health care for all patients. Unless cultural differences are taken into account, this goal cannot be accomplished. Misunderstandings can sometimes lead to misdiagnoses, as in the case of coin rubbing. Danger signals may be overlooked with a stoic Irish or Japanese patient.

The most important underlying message of this book is that cultural behavior is generally a result of adaptation to both the physical and the social environment. Different countries have different conditions—different weather, population size, vegetation, political circumstances, economic bases, and so forth. Cultures develop norms, values, and behaviors that are suited to these conditions. Over time, they take on the strength of tradition. Even when circumstances change, traditions often do not.

We are socialized by our culture at an early age. Early conditioning is very hard to overcome. Even when we move to a new country, where the customs and values are different, it is hard to change, even under the best of circumstances. Illness, particularly illness that requires hospitalization, is far from the best of circumstances. On the contrary, it is the very time when we are most likely to regress and behave in ways that were reinforced in childhood.

Certainly it is best for people to speak the language of the country in which they are living. Unfortunately, many immigrants to this country work long hours every day at physical labor. They are often too tired at night to attend English classes. Furthermore, they tend to live in ethnic communities where everyone speaks their native language, and thus they have no pressing need to learn English. Finally, not everyone has an equal facility with language. English is difficult to learn. The rules are far more irregular than in the Romance languages such as Spanish. It is much easier for children to learn new languages, perhaps because they are not so inhibited or afraid to make mistakes as adults are. For many people, the idea of learning a difficult new language may be overwhelming. So though ideally everyone in the United States should speak English, many do not. Does that mean they should receive inferior care?

Whether patients should speak English and adapt to our ways is irrelevant. The fact is that they do not and may not. The options are to provide inferior medical care (and experience high levels of stress resulting from frustration) or to make accommodations so as to provide optimal care (while at the same time reducing stress and frustration).

The anecdotes in this book were chosen to illustrate some of the most common or difficult problems that occur in hospitals as a result of cultural differences. In some instances, knowledge can prevent problems from occurring, as in the case of dietary taboos or preferences. In other cases, merely understanding why patients act the way they do may help hospital personnel be more compassionate and experience less frustration. Although at times it may appear that a patient's sole goal is to make things difficult for nurses and doctors, this is rarely the case. The patients are merely behaving in ways they were taught were appropriate or that were successful at other times in their lives.

Racism, discrimination, and prejudice are a sad reality of modern life. They usually result from stereotyping, from seeing people as members of a group, rather than as individuals. Don't perpetuate this mistake. Be sensitive to feelings of perceived racism among minority group members. As a result of years of slavery and discrimination, Blacks, for example, may be sensitive even to unintentional threats to their self-esteem.

In summary, I will highlight the important points of the eleven preceding chapters.

Communication and Time Orientation

Idioms should be avoided whenever possible. Also remember that all English is not the same. The same words may have different meanings in different English-speaking countries, for example "fanny" and "fag" (the latter is a cigarette in England). The identity of the speaker is also important. A Black person may refer to a Black man as a "boy," but it would be very inappropriate for a Caucasian to do so.

A patient should be referred to as Mr., Mrs., Miss, or Ms. unless told by the patient to do otherwise. People suffer tremendous loss of dignity when they become patients; it is important not to add unnecessarily to this loss.

Remember that "yes" may not always mean the affirmative; for an Asian, it may be a way of avoiding the embarrassment of saying "no." Or, it may be the grammatically correct but misleading answer to a negative question, as in, "Haven't you taken your medication yet today?" It is best to ask open-ended questions and to avoid negatives whenever possible. Also be aware that masculine and feminine pronouns do not exist in many Asian languages, and interpret statements accordingly.

When choosing an interpreter, it is not enough for the person to speak the same language as the patient. It is important to choose someone of the appropriate sex and relationship. Same-sex interpreters are usually best. Children and other family members are often inappropriate.

Americans do not feel as comfortable with conversational silences as do some ethnic groups. When talking to Navaho patients, be sure to give them plenty of time to respond to your questions.

People from many cultures may be reluctant to discuss anything about their personal life or problems. Hispanic patients may feel it is the business only of other family members, not strangers. Asian patients may be trying to avoid the stigma of mental illness or fearful of government reprisals. Gypsy patients may simply not trust outsiders.

Eye contact may have different meaning in different cultures. Lack of eye contact may reflect respect or concern rather than disinterest.

Realize that not everyone will be comfortable being touched. Asians usually refrain from public gestures of affection. Opposite-sex touching should be avoided with Orthodox Jews and devout Muslims.

Try not to use gestures, because many of those with neutral or even positive connotations in the United States ("okay," "thumbs up," and "victory") may have insulting or sexually suggestive connotations elsewhere.

Time orientation varies among different ethnic groups (as well as among individuals). Present-oriented individuals may be late for appointments. Tardiness may be compounded by poverty; reliance on public transportation and difficulties in getting time off from work may also contribute to this problem. In addition, people with a present time orientation may not practice preventive health care, and those with a past orientation may be reluctant to try new techniques.

Pain

Some cultures encourage emotional expressiveness while others encourage emotional control. Speak with the family to ascertain whether the individual is a typical representative of his or her culture and, if so, adjust the attention given accordingly. It is important not to ignore the stoic Asian or Irish patient and not become overly concerned with the moans of a Mediterranean or Middle Eastern patient. Since many Asians may practice traditional stoicism, they might not request pain medication. The safest approach is to anticipate their needs and simply administer the medication without waiting for a request.

Recognize that many people, particularly Filipinos and East Indians, may hold a culturally enhanced fear of addiction. In that case, it is important to discuss with them the need for pain medication, as well as the risks of addiction.

Remember that not everyone will want the least invasive forms of medication. If there are alternatives available, present them to the patient, and let the patient choose.

Religion, Beliefs, and Customs

Religion is often an integral part of people's lives, becoming even more important during times of illness. Patients' religious beliefs should be respected and incorporated into their care whenever possible. Time should be set aside for the patient to pray undisturbed, if so desired.

Try to respect religious prohibitions, such as contact with the opposite sex. In such cases, make every effort to assign same-sex caregivers.

Some religions have beliefs that conflict with Western medicine, for example, Jehovah's Witnesses' beliefs about blood transfusions. When confronted with such conflicts, consider the patients' perspective and the possibility that their beliefs may be correct. Also remember that they live within a social network. The social cost of violating religious taboos may be too high for them to be willing to do so. If patients are resistant to Western medicine because they believe only God can heal, try to incorporate their faith into your treatment.

It is also important to be aware of holy days and restrictions associated with them, such as the Orthodox Jewish prohibition against any form of work on the Sabbath (Saturday).

Recognize that sacred symbols can take many forms, from Catholic rosary beads to Cambodian wrist strings. These should not be removed without discussion, and it is best to try to keep them in contact with the patient's body whenever possible. This can be psychologically important to the patient.

People may hold magical beliefs, such as in evil eye or soul loss. Ignoring such beliefs can cause emotional stress for the patient. You need share their beliefs to respect them.

Some cultures have taboos regarding the body, such as which hand is used for various functions. Try to accommodate such practices whenever possible. Hair has significance in many cultures. It should not be shaved or cut without first discussing it with the patient. If the patient objects, alternatives should be sought.

Dietary Practices

Many religions and cultures have dietary taboos or prescriptions which should be ascertained at the intake interview. Muslims and Orthodox Jews are forbidden pork, Hindus beef, and Asians and Hispanics may be concerned about hot/cold body balance.

Different cultures have different food preferences. It should not be assumed that a patient who refuses to eat lacks an appetite; it may just be that inappropriate foods were served, or that appropriate foods were served in an inappropriate form. (Japanese, for example, usually eat meat cut into small slices and mixed with vegetables rather than in the form of a steak.) Suggest alternative foods to the patient or the family. Be aware that some ethnic groups cannot tolerate certain foods, such as dairy products, and adjust the menus accordingly. If there are restrictions to be placed upon the patient's diet after discharge, be sure to discuss them with the family members who do the cooking. Some ethnic diets are extremely high in fats and salt; alternative cooking methods will need to be learned.

Family

Most non-Anglo cultures value family highly. Many patients come from large families—a necessity in agricultural communities. When a family member is ill, the rest feel they must be there with the patient. For the well-being of the patient and the family, it is best to be as flexible as possible regarding visitors and visiting hours, setting limits when necessary. If possible, place patients with frequent large groups of visitors (such as Gypsies) in a room at the end of the hall, or where there will be minimum disturbance to other patients.

Self-care, a medical goal for patients, is often ignored. The family will often take over feeding and grooming the patient. This may be an important way for family members to demonstrate their love and respect for the patient. It may also be a way for a male patient from a hierarchical culture to demonstrate continued control over his family, despite physical weakness. If self-care is necessary for recovery—as in the case of burn patients—give the family tasks that will not impede the patient's progress. If the staff's emphasis on self-care is primarily a reflection of the American value of independence, do not insist but allow the family to continue caring for the patient.

Some families may be particularly demanding of hospital staff and services. Often, the best way to handle them is to spend a few minutes talking with them when the patient first checks in, and then a few minutes in conversation each day. Ask questions about the patient as a *person* (e.g., what kinds of things does does the patient enjoy doing? How many children are in the family?). Let them know that you care about their loved one. Also, offer the family small, helpful tasks they can do, such as rubbing lotion onto the patient's hands, so they feel they are doing something useful. It is often the feeling of helplessness that causes them to be demanding.

Recognize that although it may be against hospital policy, many patients will try to give gifts to nurses, either to remove the debt of obligation or to ensure good service. It is best to accept such gifts but to encourage only those that can be shared by the entire nursing staff.

Realize that kinship systems may differ from that found among Anglo Americans and that other relatives may be closer to a child than the biological parents. Hospital rules regarding who may sign informed consent will still have to be followed, but consult with appropriate relatives, such as grandparents or uncles, for example, in the case of a Navaho or African patient.

Men and Women

Few cultures share an egalitarian ideal for men and women. In most cultures, men are thought to be the heads of the house and the primary decision makers. This situation is gradually changing as a result of the spread of Western influence, but change is slow and sporadic. Males may therefore serve as spokespersons for their wives. Female caregivers should remember that these wives may be perfectly content with the arrangement.

In hierarchical cultures, age generally carries authority. Elders may make decisions for their grown children. Often it may be the best policy for hospital personnel to address their first remarks to the eldest family member present, rather than to the patient.

Some cultures, such as Asian or Middle Eastern, may prefer male children over females because males traditionally take care of parents when they are old, and they carry on the family name. The latter is especially important in cultures like Chinese that practice ancestor worship. Although hospital staff may be disturbed at seeing parents show preference for male children, they should not expect people to change.

Female purity is especially important in the Middle East and in Muslim countries in general. Intimate contact between the sexes is forbidden outside of marriage. The use of same-sex doctors and nurses will get the best results. Modesty is also a major concern in Hispanic, Asian, and Gypsy cultures; in fact, it is important in most cultures and should be respected. Although it is often not expedient to take the time to ensure a patient's personal privacy, it is a goal to strive for with all patients.

If you have any female patients who are "circumcised," do not act in a judgmental manner, but you might discuss with them the health and legal consequences of infibulation during health teaching so they can make informed choices for their own daughters.

Staff Relations

A major source of conflict between staff members derives from the fact that in many other cultures the power gap between doctors and nurses is much greater than in the United States. This gap is exacerbated by the fact that many physicians and nurses come from hierarchically based countries, such as those in Asia, India, and the Middle East, where men are perceived as more important than women. Thus, many foreign-born male doctors are exceedingly domineering and often find themselves in confrontations with American-born nurses.

There are two ways to approach this problem. One is for hospitals to offer in-service training to foreign-born doctors on what to expect from American nurses. The fact that an important function of nurses is to act as patient advocate prevents them from blindly obeying any order the physician gives if they feel it may be detrimental to the patient. Physicians often interpret that as the nurse disobeying and disrespecting the doctor, rather than standing up for the patient. Another approach is to suggest that nurses, realizing that the physician may be unaware of the American health care system, act in a less confrontational manner.

The power gap between doctors and nurses in other countries also creates a problem for foreign-born nurses, particularly those from countries in which women are socialized to be submissive. Many, when they first come to the United States, act in a very subservient manner toward physicians and others above them in the hospital hierarchy. This can cause stress between foreign born and American-born nurses as well as impede the former's move up the nursing hierarchy, since they may lack the assertiveness skills necessary for supervisory positions. In such cases, assertiveness training classes may help, although those whose basic nature is assertive may quickly overcome their early socialization without the aid of instruction. Those who are passive both by nature and training may have to be content with positions more suited to their temperament.

The lack of sexual equality in some countries encourages male employees to refuse to take orders from a female supervisor. While this behavior may have to be tolerated in patients, termination is an option if change does not follow open discussion of the problem with staff.

Several other problems can arise between foreign-born and American-born nurses. The role of the American nurse is often much broader than that of the foreign-born caregiver. Not only must the nurse take care of the patient's health needs but also provide personal and psychosocial care—functions usually handled by the family in other countries. A foreign-born nurse's reluctance do such things may be interpreted as laziness or bad nursing. Similarly, some foreign-born nurses may feel that asking for or accepting help from another nurse is a sign that he or she cannot do the job, creating conflict between co-workers, who perceive instead that the individual is not a "team player." Many of these misunderstandings could be resolved by an in-service workshop on the specific jobs expected of American nurses as well as the nature of nursing culture.

Since the role of the doctor vis-à-vis the patient is so different in the United States, where patients often want to be listened to and actively participate in their treatment, it can be problematical for foreign-born physicians who believe the authority of the doctor precludes the need to explain anything to the patient. At the same time, patients who come from some Asian and Native American cultures may expect physicians to act more authoritatively, neither asking questions nor revealing serious diagnoses. This can prove tricky for doctors, on legal as well as social grounds. One suggestion, again, is in-service training on doctor/patient roles in different cultures. Sometimes, it might be best for the nurse to ask questions of the patient. Generally, some sensitivity on the part of physicians, and discussion with family members, will be effective.

Other problems which frequently arise between staff members involve language and communication. Speaking native languages in the workplace is a very sore point at many hospitals. The best approach to handling this problem is twofold. First, there should be open discussion among both sides, each sharing their feelings and reasons for their behavior or attitude. Second, there should be clear rules: no speaking in a foreign language around patients, switch to English when non-native speakers enter the room, but allow it on break time when no non-speakers are around.

Other language problems, which frequently arise with speakers of Asian languages, can be avoided with knowledge of different language customs and social rules. People need to let each other know, in a friendly way, when something someone said has hurt them in some way. Such misunderstandings are often culturally based and can be cleared up immediately.

Finally, hospital staff may have religious beliefs that interfere with some medical practices, as in the case of a Catholic nurse who refused to assist in an abortion. Staff members should make such restrictions known to their supervisors, who in turn should try to respect them.

Birth

Though birth is a universal event, behavior during labor is strongly culturally conditioned. Women are taught to be loud or stoic, to push or not push during different times. Generally, cultures that value emotional expressiveness allow or encourage expressiveness during labor; those that value emotional control encourage stoicism during labor. Labor is not a time to try to change patients' behavior. If possible, women with similar levels of expressiveness should be put in the same room.

Labor attendants also vary cross-culturally. One should not assume that a woman's husband is the desired labor partner. In many cultures, including Asian and Hispanic, the woman's mother may be more appropriate. This matter can easily be discussed with the patient.

Many cultures practice a postpartum lying-in period during which time bathing and exercise are prohibited. Certain foods must be avoided while others are encouraged. Though with current Diagnostic Related Groups new mothers are rarely in the hospital long enough for this to be an issue, it should be taken into account, particularly with Asian, East Indian, and Hispanic women. Also try to avoid offering ice water, unless it is requested, because it may be thought to be too cold for a body that has just been depleted of heat through the process of giving birth. Be aware that young mothers may be willing to comply with Western medical recommendations but hesitate to do so in the presence of their more traditional mothers.

Bonding between mother and child is often a concern. Some cultures, such as Vietnamese, may appear to have bonding problems because of beliefs that spirits want to steal newborns. An apparent lack of attention may actually be an effort to thwart the interest of spirits. Health care professionals should follow the lead of the parents in their own displays of attention to infants. In many cultures, babies are not formally named until up to a month after the birth. This custom should be respected and not viewed as evidence of lack of bonding. Apparent neglect may also be a part of the lying-in period. Among East Indians, for example, family members take over the care of the infant to allow the new mother time to recuperate.

Women from various cultures may wait several days before breastfeeding their newborns so as to allow their milk to come in. Since the early colostrum is important to the infant's health, patient education may be necessary to encourage early breastfeeding.

Realize that husbands and wives may have different desires regarding family size and be sensitive to this in discussions of birth control and sterilization.

Death and Dying

American culture values autonomy; a great deal of emphasis is placed on the patient's "right to know." This is not the case in many other cultures, where both the family and the patient may try to shield each other from knowledge of the seriousness of the patient's condition. When a patient enters the hospital, it would be wise to talk with a family member to discuss who should be given information about the patient's condition. If it is not the patient, the patient can then sign a waiver to that effect. At the same time, nurses should be sensitive to the needs of the patients, who may not have anyone else with whom openly to discuss their feelings about dying.

Whether or not to remove life support is a traumatic personal issue for anyone. Cultural and religious factors contribute to the decision-making process. Many of these factors, such as faith in God to perform a miracle and the desire to show faith and courage in the face of suffering, are almost predictable. Sometimes, however, they can be surprising, as in the case of the Vietnamese family who used astrology to determine the most auspicious date for their son's death.

Individuals express grief in a variety of different ways. Culture can influence whether the mourners stoically suppress their feelings or give open expression to them. The latter can create a disturbance on the floor, which can be distressing to other patients. In such cases, it would be best to move the deceased and the family to a private area, such as the chapel, so they can be allowed to grieve without disturbing other patients.

If you have Gypsy patients, realize that it is customary for them to light candles around the bed of a dying patient. Take precautions with regard to oxygen equipment.

Numbers may have lucky or unlucky associations, which should be taken into account when assigning rooms. Try to avoid use of the number 4 with Chinese and Japanese patients, since it signifies "death." Use it instead with Navaho patients since for them, it has positive connotations.

Finally, be familiar with religious and ethnic customs regarding organ donation and autopsies, and be sensitive to the patients' desires.

Mental Health

Behavior which is seen as normal in one culture may be interpreted as deviant in another; not all "deviant" behavior may be a result of mental illness, but rather an expression of cultural traits. For example, in many cultures, visions of the recently deceased are common and normal; they should not be interpreted as signs of mental illness in the absence of other symptoms.

Many people believe in the reality of what most Americans would term the "supernatural." Regardless of your own beliefs, remember that it is generally more effective to treat problems from within the context of the individual's world view. For example, use exorcism to treat possession. Incorporate traditional healers when possible.

Realize that it may be extremely difficult to get members of some ethnic groups to talk about personal problems due to the highly stigmatized nature of mental illness or the belief that personal problems should remain within the family. Utilize the aid of trusted traditional healers or more acculturated family members when necessary.

Finally, be especially alert for stress caused by inter-cultural conflict among the children of immigrants. They may require the help of culturally aware social workers, though any mention of "counseling" or "mental illness" should generally be avoided.

Folk Medicine

All cultures have developed their own methods for treating illness based on observed cause-and-effect relationships. Some techniques, such as coin rubbing and cupping, produce marks that may appear to be signs of child abuse or unrelated symptoms. It is important to recognize these before jumping to unwarranted conclusions.

Conventional wisdom generally treats fever by trying to sweat it out; Western medicine tries to cool it down. Patients may be very resistant to cooling measures. When such measures are used, the rationale for them should be carefully explained. First, however, consider the possibility that allowing the patient to have additional blankets may have an important psychological effect.

Patients may occasionally experience pica—a craving for nonfood substances. A common pica among pregnant Black women is Argo laundry starch. The quantity consumed should be monitored for health reasons, but the psychological benefits of allowing a small amount may be substantial.

When doctors are unable to cure a patient or to obtain consent to certain procedures, it may be beneficial to agree to a patient's request to bring in a traditional healer. Such healers are occasionally successful, whether from the efficaciousness of their treatments or a placebo effect.

Noncompliance regarding medications may result from such things as unfamiliarity with the prescription system or a conflict in time orientation. Taking the time carefully to explain procedures and reasons for the medication will usually avoid the problem.

Body image varies cross-culturally. "Beauty is in the eye of the beholder" is an old cliché but an accurate one nonetheless. Members of some cultures may value features Americans dislike, for example, scars or body fat. Do not assume that everyone shares our ideals. Fat may be seen as a sign of health and fertility in a culture where starvation and malnutrition are common.

Finally, remember that all toilets are not alike and that bathroom habits may vary. People from Third World and even some European countries may be used to squatting over a hole and may have difficulty using a toilet seat or bedpan.

Summary

Transcultural health care requires a holistic and culturally relativistic approach. Treat the patient as a whole person with psychological and spiritual needs as well as physical ones. See patients as members of a family unit, not as just individuals. Do not assume that patients or co-workers will view the world the same way that you do; they may have different values and different ways of looking at things. Do not make assumptions and do respect differences. Recognize that other people's views are just as valid as yours.

If this advice were applied to all patients, no matter what their ethnic or cultural background, we would go a long way toward providing better care for patients from all cultures.

Finally, one of the most effective things a culturally diverse hospital can do is encourage the staff to talk openly to each other about their cultures. The cultures of the patient population are usually well-represented by the staff population. Ask questions about behaviors that disturb you; the answers may be surprising. A trained facilitator may be necessary to start such discussions, but once people see that it is "safe" to ask questions, an open dialogue should continue on its own. Individuals must be willing to let others know (in a friendly manner) when someone has done something which offends them, and, at the same time, "lighten up" a bit and realize that most people are offensive out of ignorance and not because they intentionally want to hurt others.

Imagine what would happen if everyone followed this advice everywhere, on the streets as well as in the hospital.

Selected Bibliography

GENERAL

Anderson, R. (1996) *Magic, Science, and Health.* New York: Harcourt Brace College Publishers.

Andrews, M. M., and J. S. Boyle. (1995) *Transcultural Concepts in Nursing Care.* 2d ed. Boston: Scott, Foresman.

Bauwens, E., ed. (1978) *The Anthropology of Health.* St. Louis: C. V. Mosby.

Berlin, E. A., and W. C. Fowkes, Jr. (1983) A teaching framework for cross-cultural health care: Application in family practice. *Western Journal of Medicine* 139: 928–933.

Branch, M. F., and P. P. Paxton. (1976) *Providing Safe Nursing Care for Ethnic People of Color.* New York: Appleton-Century-Crofts.

Brink, P. J. (1976) *Transcultural Nursing: A Book of Readings.* Englewood Cliffs, NJ: Prentice-Hall.

Brownlee, A. T. (1978) *Community, Culture and Care: A Cross Cultural Guide for Healthworkers.* St. Louis: C. V. Mosby.

Bullough, B., and V. L. Bullough. (1972) *Poverty, Ethnic Identity and Health Care.* New York: Appleton-Century-Crofts.

Bullough, V. L., and B. Bullough. (1982) *Health Care for Other Americans.* New York: Appleton-Century-Crofts.

Campinha-Bacote, Josepha. (1994) *The Process of Cultural Competence in Health Care: A Culturally Competent Model of Care.* 2d ed. Wyoming, OH: Transcultural C.A.R.E. Associates.

Chrisman, N. (1991) Culture-sensitive nursing care. In M. Patrick, S. Woods, R. Craven, J. Rokosky, and P. Bruno, eds., *Medical-Surgical Nursing: Pathophysiological Concepts,* 2d ed., pp. 34–46. New York: J. B. Lippincott.

Chrisman, N. (1991) Cultural systems. In S. Baird, R. McCorkle, and M. Grant, eds., *Cancer Nursing: A Comprehensive Textbook.* Philadelphia: W.B. Saunders Co.

Clark, M. M. (1983) Cultural context of medical practice. *Western Journal of Medicine* 139(6): 806–810.

Elling, R. H. (1977) *Socio-Cultural Influences on Health and Health Care.* New York: Springer.

Elliott, J. L. (1972) Cultural barriers to the utilization of health services. *Inquiry* 9: 28–35.

Foster, G. M., and B. G. Anderson. (1978) *Medical Anthropology.* New York: John Wiley & Sons.

Gorrie, M. (1989) Reaching clients through cross cultural education. *Journal of Gerontological Nursing* 15(10): 29–31.

Hahn, R. A. (1995) *Sickness and Healing: An Anthropological Perspective.* New Haven, CT: Yale University Press.

Hartog, J., and E. A. Hartog. (1983) Cultural aspects of health and illness behavior in hospitals. *Western Journal of Medicine* 139: 910–916.

Harwood, A. (1981) *Ethnicity and Medical Care.* Cambridge, MA: Harvard University Press.

Henderson, G., and M. Primeaux, eds. (1981) *Transcultural Health Care.* Menlo Park, CA: Addison-Wesley.

Kavanagh, K. H., and P. H. Kennedy (1992) *Promoting Cultural Diversity: Strategies for Health Care Professionals.* Newbury Park, CA: Sage Publications.

Kim, S. S. (1983) Ethnic elders and American health care: A physician's perspective. *Western Journal of Medicine* 139: 885–891.

Klein, N., ed. (1979) *Culture, Curers & Contagion.* Novato, CA: Chandler & Sharp.

Kleinman, A., L. Eisenberg, and B. Good. (1978) Culture, illness and care: Clinical lessons. Anthropologic and cross-cultural research. *Annals of Internal Medicine* 88: 251–258.

Leininger, M. (1970) *Nursing and Anthropology: Two Worlds to Blend.* New York: John Wiley.

Leininger, M. (1978) *Transcultural Nursing: Concepts, Theories and Practices.* New York: John Wiley.

McElroy, A., and P. K. Townsend. (1989) *Medical Anthropology in Ecological Perspective.* Boulder, CO: Westview Press

Mindel, C. H., and R. W. Habenslein, eds. (1976) *Ethnic Families in America.* New York: Elsevier.

Moore, L., P. Van Arsdale, J. Glittenberg, and R. Aldrich. (1980) *The Biocultural Basis of Health.* St. Louis: C. V. Mosby.

Orque, M. S., B. Bloch, and L. S. A. Monrroy. (1983) *Ethnic Nursing Care: A Multicultural Approach.* St. Louis: C. V. Mosby.

Payer, L. (1988) *Medicine and Culture.* New York: Henry Holt.

Rackovsky, I. (1980) Nurses, nursing and culture. *Supervisor Nurse* (July): 20–22.

Read, M. (1966) *Culture, Health and Disease.* London: Tavistock.

Ruiz, M. C. J. (1981) Open-closed mindedness, intolerance of ambiguity and nursing faculty attitudes toward culturally different patients. *Nursing Research* 30(3): 177-181.

Saunders, L. (1954) *Cultural Differences and Medical Care.* New York: Sage.

Smith, S. (1989) People without land. *American Journal of Nursing* 89(2): 208–209.

Spector, R. E. (1991) *Cultural Diversity in Health and Illness.* 3d ed. Norwalk, CT: Appleton-Century-Crofts.

Spicer, E. H., ed. (1977) *Ethnic Medicine in the Southwest:* Tucson: University of Arizona Press.

Stein, H. F. (1990) *American Medicine as Culture.* Boulder, CO: Westview Press.

Valente, S. M. (1989, September) Overcoming cultural barriers. *California Nurse,* pp. 4–5.

JOURNALS

Journal of Transcultural Nursing
Medical Anthropology Quarterly
Medical Anthropology

ETHNIC GROUPS

ASIANS AND EAST INDIANS

Abu-Saad, H., J. Kayser-Jones, and J. Tien. (1982) Asian nursing students in the United States. *Journal of Nursing Education* 21 (7): 11–15.

Anderson, J. N. (1983) Health and illness in Philipino immigrants. *Western Journal of Medicine* 139: 811–819.

Bowers, J. Z. (1965) *Medical Education in Japan.* New York: Harper & Row.

Campbell, T., and B. Chang. (1981) Health care of the Chinese in America. In G. Henderson and M. Primeaux, eds., *Transcultural Health Care,* pp. 162–171. Menlo Park, CA: Addison-Wesley.

Chang, B. (1981) Asian-American patient care. In G. Henderson and M. Primeaux, eds., *Transcultural Health Care,* pp. 255–278. Menlo Park, CA: Addison-Wesley.

Chen-Louie, T. (1983) Nursing care of Chinese American patients. In M. S. Orque, B. Bloch, and L. S. A. Monrroy, eds., *Ethnic Nursing Care: A Multicultural Approach,* pp. 183–218. St. Louis: C. V. Mosby.

Clayton, J., and A. Henley. (1982) Asians in the hospital: Illness and the life cycle. *Health and Social Services Journal* (August): 972–974.

De Gracia, R. (1979) Health care of the American Asian patient. *Critical Care Update* (December): 19.

Dyck, B. (1989) The paper crane. *American Journal of Nursing* 89(6): 824–825.

Ellis, J. (1982) Southeast Asian refugees and maternity care: The Oakland experience. *Birth* 9(3): 191–194.

Gonzales, N. (1966) Filipino culture and food habits. *Philippine Journal of Nutrition* 19: 194–201.

Gordon, V. D., I. M. Matousek, and T. A. Lang. (1980) Southeast Asian refugees: Life in America. *American Journal of Nursing* 80: 2031–2036.

Grippin, J. T. (1979) The Japanese American client. *Issues in Mental Health Nursing* 2: 57–69.

Hashizume, S., and J. Takano. (1983) Nursing care of Japanese American patients. In M. S. Orque, B. Bloch, and L. S. A. Monrroy, eds., *Ethnic Nursing Care: A Multicultural Approach,* pp. 219–243. St. Louis: C. V. Mosby.

Henderson, L. (1967) *Vietnam and Countries of the Mekong.* Camden, NJ: Thomas Nelson and Sons.

Hollingsworth, A., P. L. Brown, and D. A. Brooten. (1980) The refugees and childbearing: What to expect. *RN Magazine* 43: 45–48.

Kiefer, C. W. (1974) *Changing Cultures, Changing Lives: An Ethnographic Study of Three Generations of Japanese Americans.* San Francisco: Jossey-Bass.

Kitano, H. (1969) *Japanese-Americans.* Englewood Cliffs, NJ: Prentice-Hall.

Kleinman, A., P. Kunstader, E. R. Alexander, and J. Gale, eds. (1975) *Medicine in Chinese Cultures.* Washington, DC: Fogarty International Center.

Kuhni, C. Q. (1990) When cultures clash at the bedside. *RN* (January): 23–26.

Landry, L. (1968) *The Land and People of Southeast Asia.* New York: J. B. Lippincott.

LeBar, F. and A. Suddard. (1960) *Laos: Its People, Its Society, Its Culture.* New Haven, CT: HRAF Press.

Lebra, T. S., and W. P. Lebra. (1974) *Japanese Culture and Behavior.* Honolulu: University of Hawaii Press.

Lee, R. (1970) *Chinese in America.* Hong Kong: Hong Kong University Press.

Leslie, C., ed. (1976) *Asian Medical Systems.* Los Angeles: University of California Press.

Leyn, R. B. (1978) The challenge of caring for child refugees from Southeast Asia. *American Journal of Maternal Child Nursing* 3: 178–182.

Liu, W. T., M. Lamanna, and A. Muralta. (1979) *Transition to Nowhere: Vietnamese Refugees in America.* Nashville, TN: Charter House.

Lock, M. (1983) Japanese responses to social change: Making the strange familiar. *Western Journal of Medicine* 139: 829–834.

Longo, B. (1990) Confusing blend of Asian, U.S. medicine. *NURSEweek* (February 5): 1, 22.

Muecke, M. A. (1983) In search of healers: Southeast Asian refugees in the American health care system. *Western Journal of Medicine* 129: 835–840.

Ohnuki-Tierney, E. (1984) *Illness and Culture in Contemporary Japan.* New York: Cambridge University Press.

Orque, M. S. (1983) Nursing care of Filipino American patients. In M. S. Orque, B. Bloch, and L. S. A. Monrroy, eds., *Ethnic Nursing Care: A Multicultural Approach,* pp. 149–181. St. Louis: C. V. Mosby.

Orque, M. S. (1983) Nursing care of South Vietnamese patients. In M. S. Orque, R. Bloch, and L. S. A. Monrroy, eds., *Ethnic Nursing Care: A Multicultural Approach,* pp. 245–270. St. Louis: C. V. Mosby.

Osgood, C. (1954) *The Koreans and Their Culture.* Tokyo: Houghton Mifflin.

Rairdan, B., and Z. Higgs. (1992) When your patient is a Hmong refugee. *American Journal of Nursing* 25 : 52–55.

Ramakrishna, J. (1992) Health, illness, and immigration: East Indians in the United States. *Western Journal of Medicine* 157(3): 265–270.

Schacht, R. (1989) Epilogue: Glimpses of China and Chinese elders. *Journal of Gerontological Nursing* 15(1): 39–40.

Sheppard, H. (1990) How Hispanic cultural patterns affect care-givers. *NURSEweek,* (February 5): 15–16.

Sung, B. L. (1989) Bicultural conflict. In E. Angeloni, ed., *Annual Editions, Anthropology 89/90,* pp. 228–235. Guilford, CT: Dushkin.

Tsung-Yi, L. (1983) Psychiatry and Chinese culture. *Western Journal of Medicine* 139: 862–867.

Wilson, D. K. (1980) The refugee. *RN Magazine,* (November): 42–48.

Wolf, M. (1968) *Women in Chinese Society.* New York: Appleton-Century-Crofts.

BLACKS

Billingsley, A. (1968) *Black Families in White America.* Englewood Cliffs, NJ: Prentice-Hall.

Billingsley, A. (1974) *Black Families and the Struggle for Survival.* New York: Friendship Press.

Burgess, H. A. (1987) Into the Sudan. *American Journal of Nursing* 87(7): 927–929.

Harrison, I. E., and D. S. Harrison. (1971) The Black family experience and health behavior. In C. Crawford, ed., *Health and the Family.* New York: Macmillan.

Jones, E. L. (1976) Nursing care of the Black patient. In D. Luckraft, ed., *Black Awareness: Implications for Black Patient Care,* pp. 36–37. New York: American Journal of Nursing.

Lewis, D. K. (1975) The black family socialization and sex roles. *Phylon* 36: 221–237.

Luckraft, D., ed. (1976) *Black Awareness: Implications for Black Patient Care.* New York: American Journal of Nursing.

Martin, E. P., and J. M. Martin. (1978) *The Black Extended Family*. Chicago: University of Chicago Press.

Mays, R. M. (1979) Primary health care and the Black family. *Nurse Practitioner* 4: 13.

Meindl, N., and C. Getty. (1981) Life-styles of Black families headed by women. In C. Getty and W. Humphreys, eds., *Understanding the Family*, pp. 157–184. New York: Appleton-Century-Crofts.

Nobles, W. W., and G. M. Nobles. (1976) African roots in Black families: The social-psychological dynamics of Black family life and the implications for nursing care. In D. Luckraft, ed., *Black Awareness: Implications for Black Patient Care*, p. 19. New York: American Journal of Nursing.

Parker, S., and R. J. Kleiner, eds. (1966) *Mental Illness in the Urban Negro Community*. New York: Free Press.

Parsons, T., and K. B. Clark. (1965) *The Negro American*. Boston: Beacon Press.

Seham, M. (1973) *Blacks and American Medical Care*. Minneapolis: University of Minnesota Press.

Snow, L. F. (1977) Popular medicine in a Black neighborhood. In E. H. Spicer, ed., *Ethnic Medicine in the Southwest*, pp. 19–95. Tucson: University of Arizona Press.

Snow, L. F. (1983) Traditional health beliefs and practices among lower class Black Americans. *Western Journal of Medicine* 139: 820–828.

Snow, L. F. (1993) *Walkin' over Medicine*. Boulder, CO: Westview Press.

Thomas, D. N. (1981) Black American patient care. In G. Henderson and M. Primeaux, eds., *Transcultural Health Care*. Menlo Park, CA: Addison-Wesley.

Ullendorf, E. (1960) *The Ethiopians*. London: Oxford University Press.

White, E. (1974) Health and the Black person: An annotated bibliography. *American Journal of Nursing* 74: 1839–1841.

Williams, R. A. (1975) *Textbook of Black Related Diseases*. New York: McGraw-Hill.

GYPSIES

Anderson, G., and B. Tighe. (1979) Gypsy culture and health care. In N. Klein ed., *Culture, Curers & Contagion*, pp. 195–200. Novato, CA: Chandler & Sharp.

Brink, S. (1988) Doctoring Gypsies. *Boston Magazine* 7: 80–86.

Clark, M. W. (1967) Vanishing vagabonds: The American Gypsies. *Texas Quarterly* 10: 204–210.

Clebert, J. P. (1969) *The Gypsies*. Baltimore: Penguin.

Cohn, W. (1973) *The Gypsies*. Reading, MA: Addison-Wesley.

Gropper, R. C. (1975) *Gypsies in the City*. Princeton, NJ: Darwin Press.

Kephart, W. M. (1989) The Gypsies. In E. Angeloni, ed., *Annual Editions: Anthropology 89/90*, pp. 122–137. Guilford, CT: Dushkin.

Manneli, F. (1974) Gypsies, culture, and child care. *Pediatrics* 54(5): 603–607.

Sutherland, A. (1975) *Gypsies: The Hidden Americans*. New York: Free Press.

Sutherland, A. (1992) Gypsies and health care. *Western Journal of Medicine* 157(3): 276–280.

Sway, M. (1988) *Familiar Strangers: Gypsy Life in America*. Champaign: University of Illinois Press.

Webb, G. E. C. (1960) *Gypsies: The Secret People*. London: Herbert Jenkins.

Yoors, J. (1967) *Gypsies*. New York: Simon and Schuster.

HISPANICS

Baca, J. E. (1978) Some health beliefs of the Spanish speaking. In R. A. Martinez, ed., *Hispanic Culture and Health Care*, pp. 92–98. St. Louis: C. V. Mosby.

Barnett, S. E. (1980) Migrant health revisited: A model for statewide health planning and services. *American Journal of Public Health* 70: 1092–1094.

Burma, J. H., ed. (1970) *Mexican Americans in the United States*. Cambridge, MA: Schenkman.

Clark, M. (1959) *Health in the Mexican-American Culture*. Los Angeles: University of California Press.

Delgado, M., and D. Humm-Delgado. (1982) Natural support systems: Source of strength in Hispanic communities. *Social Work* 27: 83–89.

Diaz-Guerrero, R. (1955) Neurosis and the Mexican family structure. *American Journal of Psychiatry* 112: 411–417.

Grebler, L., J. W. Moore, and R. G. Guzman. (1970) *The Mexican-American People: The Nation's Second Largest Minority*. New York: Free Press.

Kay, M. A. (1977) Health and illness in a Mexican American barrio. In E. H. Spicer, ed., *Ethnic Medicine in the Southwest*. Tucson: University of Arizona Press.

Keefe, S., A. Padilla, and M. Carlos. (1979) The Mexican-American family as an emotional support system. *Human Organization* 38: 144–152.

Madsen, W. (1964) *The Mexican-Americans of South Texas*. New York: Holt, Rinehart & Winston.

Martinez, R. A., ed. (1978) *Hispanic Culture and Health Care*. St. Louis: C. V. Mosby.

Mindel, C. (1980) Extended familism among urban Mexican Americans, Anglos and Blacks. *Hispanic Journal of Behavioral Sciences* 2: 21–34.

Monrroy, L. (1983) Nursing care of Raza/Latina patients. In M. S. Orque, B. Bloch, and L. Monrroy, eds., *Ethnic Nursing Care: A Multicultural Approach*, pp. 115–148. St. Louis: C. V. Mosby.

Murillo, N. (1978) The Mexican American Family. In R. A. Martinez, ed., *Hispanic Culture and Health Care*, pp. 3–18. St. Louis: C. V. Mosby.

Murillo-Rohde, I. (1981) Hispanic American patient care. In G. Henderson and M. Primeaux, eds., *Transcultural Health Care*, pp. 224–238. Menlo Park, CA: Addison-Wesley.

Nall, F. C., and J. Speilberg. (1967) Social and cultural factors in the responses of Mexican-Americans to medical treatment. *Journal of Health and Social Behavior* 8: 299–308.

Ramirez, S., and R. Parres. (1957) Some dynamic patterns in the organization of the Mexican family. *International Journal of Social Psychiatry* 3: 18–21.

Rubel, A. (1960) Concepts of disease in Mexican-American culture. *American Anthropologist* 62: 795–814.

Samora, J. (1978) Conception of health and disease among Spanish Americans. In R. Martinez, ed., *Hispanic Culture and Health Care*, pp. 65–74. St. Louis: C. V. Mosby.

Saunders, L. (1954) *Cultural Differences and Medical Care: The Case of the Spanish-Speaking People of the Southwest*. New York: Russell Sage Foundation.

Sharff, J. W. (1989) Free enterprise and the ghetto family. In E. Angeloni, ed., *Annual Editions: Anthropology 89/90*, pp. 117–121. Guilford, CT: Dushkin.

Sheppard, H. (1990) Hispanic culture. *NURSEweek* (Feb. 5).

Steiner, S. (1969) *La Raza: The Mexican Americans*. New York: Harper & Row.

Teichner, V. J., J. J. Cadden, and G. W. Berry. (1981) The Puerto Rican patient: Some historical, cultural and psychosocial aspects. *Journal of the American Academy of Psychoanalysis* 9: 177–189.

Wagley, C. (1968) *The Latin American Tradition.* New York: Columbia University Press.

MIDDLE EASTERNERS

Berger, M. (1962) *The Arab World Today.* Garden City, NY: Doubleday.

Brooks, G. (1995) *Nine Parts of Desire.* New York: Anchor Books.

Collins, R. O., and R. L. Tignor. (1967) *Egypt and the Sudan.* Englewood Cliffs, NJ: Prentice-Hall.

Eickelman, D. F. (1981) *The Middle East: An Anthropological Approach.* Englewood Cliffs, NJ: Prentice-Hall.

Fernea, E. W. and R. A. Fernea. (1989) A look behind the veil. In E. Angeloni, ed., *Annual Editions: Anthropology 89/90*, pp. 149–153. Guilford, CT: Dushkin.

Fitzsimmons, T., ed., (1959) *Saudi Arabia: Its People, Its Society, Its Culture.* New Haven, CT: HRAF Press.

Gibb, H. A. R. (1962) *Mohammedanism.* 2d ed. New York: Oxford University Press.

Goldschmidt, A. (1979) *A Concise History of the Middle East.* Boulder, CO: Praeger.

Good, B. J. (1977) The heart of what's the matter: The semantics of illness in Iran. *Culture, Medicine, & Psychiatry* 1: 25–28.

Haim, S. G., and Kedouri, E. (1980) *Towards a Modern Iran: Studies in Thought, Politics and Society.* London: Frank Cass.

Julali, B. (1982) Iranian families. In M. McGoldrick, ed., *Ethnicity and Family Therapy*, pp. 289–302. New York: Guilford Press.

Lipson, J. G., and A. I. Meleis. (1983) Issues in health care of Middle Eastern patients. *Western Journal of Medicine* 139: 854–861.

Luna, L. (1989) Transcultural nursing care of Arab Muslims. *Journal of Transcultural Nursing* 1(1): 22–26.

Luna, L. (1994) Care and cultural context of Lebanese Muslim immigrants with Leininger's theory. *Journal of Transcultural Nursing* 5(2): 12–20.

Mansfield, P., ed., (1980) *The Middle East.* 3d ed. New York: Oxford University Press.

Meleis, A. (1981) The Arab American in the health care system. *American Journal of Nursing* 81(6): 1180–1183.

Mills, A. C. (1986) Saudi Arabia: An overview of nursing and health care. *Focus on Critical Care* 13(1): 50–56.

Nicholls, P. H. (1989) Transplanted to Saudi Arabia. *American Journal of Nursing* 89(8): 1048–1050.

Parker, J. G. (1994) The lived experience of Native Americans with diabetes within a transcultural nursing perspective. *Journal of Transcultural Nursing* 6(1): 5–11.

Patai, R. (1959) *Sex and Family in the Bible and the Middle East.* New York: Doubleday.

Patai, R. (1969) *Society, Culture and Change in the Middle East.* 3d ed. New York: Flecker.

Patai, R. (1973) *The Arab Mind.* New York: Scribner's.

Pliskin, K. L. (1992) Dysphoria and somatization in Iranian culture. *Western Journal of Medicine* 157(3): 295–300.

Shiloh, A. (1968) The interaction between the Middle Eastern and Western systems of medicine. *Social Science Medicine* 2: 235–248.

Simpson-Hebert, M. (1989) Women, food and hospitality in Iranian society. In E. Angeloni, ed., *Annual Editions: Anthropology 89/90*, pp. 154–158. Guilford, CT: Dushkin.

Stasio, M. (1989) Between two worlds. In E. Angeloni, ed., *Annual Editions: Anthropology 89/90*, pp. 159–162. Guilford, CT: Dushkin.

Wilber, D. N. (1976) *Iran, Past and Present.* Princeton, NJ: Princeton University Press.

NATIVE AMERICANS

Adair, J., and K. W. Deuschle. (1970) *The People's Health.* New York: Appleton-Century-Crofts.

Bozof, R. P. (1972) Some Navaho attitudes toward available medical care. *American Journal of Public Health* 62: 1620–1624.

Coulehan, J. H. (1980) Navaho Indian medicine: Implications for healing. *Journal of Family Practice* 10: 55–61.

Dajer, T. (1989, July) Medicine man. *Discover*, pp. 47–51.

Dennis, W. (1972) *The Hopi Child.* New York: Arno Press.

Driver, H. E. (1969) *Indians of North Americn.* Chicago: University of Chicago Press.

Edwards, E. D., and M. E. Edwards. (1980) American Indians: Working with individuals and groups. *Social Casework* 61(8): 498–506.

Hammerschlag, C. A. (1988) *The Dancing Healers: A Doctor's Journey of Healing with Native Americans.* San Francisco: Harper & Row.

Jewell, D. P. (1979) A case of a "psychotic" Navaho Indian male. In N. Klein ed., *Culture, Curers & Contagion*, pp. 155–165. Novato, CA: Chandler & Sharp.

Joe, J., C. Gallerito, and J. Pino. (1976) Cultural health traditions: American Indian perspectives. In M. Branch and P. Paxton, eds., *Providing Safe Nursing Care to Ethnic People of Color*, pp. 81–98. New York: Appleton-Century-Crofts.

Kramer, B. J. (1992) Health and aging of urban American Indians. *Western Journal of Medicine* 157(3): 281–285.

Kniep-Hardy, M., and M. A. Burkhardt. (1977) Nursing the Navaho. *American Journal of Nursing* 77: 95–96.

Kuttner, R. E., and A. B. Lorincz. (1967) Alcoholism and addiction in urbanized Sioux Indians. *Mental Hygiene* 51: 530–542.

McNickle, K. (1968) The sociocultural setting of Indian life. *American Journal of Psychiatry* (August): 115–119.

Pratson, F. J. (1970) *Land of the Four Directions.* Old Greenwich, CT: Chatham Press.

Primeaux, M. (1977) Caring for the American Indian patient. *American Journal of Nursing* 77: 91–94.

Primeaux, M., and G. Henderson. (1981) American Indian patient care. In G. Henderson and M. Primeaux, eds., *Transcultural Health Care*, pp. 239–254. Menlo Park, CA: Addison-Wesley.

Stone, E. (1962) *Medicine Among the American Indians.* New York: Hafner.

Vogel, V. J. (1981) American Indian medicine. In G. Henderson and M. Primeaux, eds., *Transcultural Health Care*, pp. 239–254. Menlo Park, CA: Addison-Wesley.

Wilson, U. M. (1983) Nursing care of American Indian patients. In M. S. Orque,

B. Bloch, and L. S. A. Monrroy, eds., *Ethnic Nursing Care: A Multicultural Approach*, pp. 271–295. St. Louis: C. V. Mosby.

Yukl, T. A., and R. Klein. (1976) Thoughts and observations on innovation of an Indian clinic in the emergency ward at Massachusetts General Hospital. *Association of American Indian Physicians* (August): 10–12.

SPECIAL TOPICS

BIRTH

Affonso, D. D. (1978) The Filipino American. In A. L. Clark, ed., *Culture, Childbearing and Health Professionals*. Philadelphia: F. A. Davis.

Bushnell, J. M. (1981) Northwest Coast American Indians' beliefs about childbirth. *Issues in Health Care of Women* 3(4): 249–261.

Clark, A. L., ed. (1978) *Culture, Childbearing and Health Professionals*. Philadelphia: F. A. Davis.

Darabi, K. F., and V. Ortiz. (1987) Childbearing among young Latino women in the U.S. *American Journal of Public Health* 77(1): 25–28.

Farris, L. S. (1976) Approaches to caring for the American Indian maternity patient. *American Journal of Maternal Child Nursing* 1(2): 82–87.

Gaviria, M., G. Stern, and S. L. Schensul. (1982) Sociocultural factors and perinatal health in a Mexican-American community. *Journal of the National Medical Association* 74(10): 983–989.

Gibbs, C. E., H. W. Martin, and M. Gutierrez. (1974) Patterns of reproductive health care among the poor of San Antonio, Texas. *American Journal of Public Health* 64: 37–40.

Hallmark, G., and M. Findlay. (1982) Cesarean birth in the operating room. *AORN Journal* 36: 978–984.

Holck, S. E., C . W. Warren, L. Morris, and R. W. Rochat. (1982) Need for family planning services among Anglo and Hispanic women in U.S. counties bordering Mexico. *Family Planning Perspectives* 14(3): 155–159.

Hollingsworth, A., L. Brown, and D. Broaten. (1980) The refugees and childbearing: What to expect. *RN Magazine* 43: 45–48.

Hook, E. B. (1978) Dietary cravings and aversions during pregnancy. *American Journal of Clinical Nutrition* 31: 1355–1362.

Horn, B. M. (1981) Cultural concepts and postpartal care. *Nursing and Health Care* 2(9): 516–517, 526–527.

Jimenez, M. H., and N. Newton. (1979) Activity and work during pregnancy and the postpartum period: A cross-cultural study of 202 societies. *American Journal of Obstetrics and Gynecology* 135(2): 171–176.

Johnston, M. (1980) Cultural variations in professional and parenting patterns. *JOGN Nursing* 9: 9–13.

Jordan, B. (1978) The cross-cultural comparison of birthing systems: Towards a biosocial analysis. In B. Jordan, ed., *Birth in Four Cultures*, pp. 32–65. St. Albans, VT: Eden Press Women's Publications.

Kay, M. A., ed. (1982) *Anthropology of Human Birth*. Philadelphia: F. A. Davis.

Kitzinger, S. (1977) Challenges in antenatal education. *Nursing Mirror* 144: 19–22.

Mead, M., and N . Newton. (1967) Cultural patterning of perinatal behavior. In S. A. Richardson and A. F. Guttmacher, eds., *Childbearing: Its Social and Psychological Aspects*, pp. 142–243. Baltimore: Williams & Wilkins.

Meleis, A. I., and L. Sorrell. (1981) Bridging cultures: Arab American women and their birth experiences. *Maternal Child Nursing* 6: 171–176.

Minkler, D. H. (1983) The role of a community-based satellite clinic in the peri-natal care of non-English speaking immigrants. *Western Journal of Medicine* 139: 905–909.

Pillsbury, B. (1982) "Doing the month": Confinement and convalescence of Chinese women after childbirth. In M. A. Kay, ed., *Anthropology of Human Birth*, pp. 119–146. Philadelphia: F. A. Davis.

Rasbridge, L. A., and J. C. Kulig. (1995) Infant feeding among Cambodian refugees. *Maternal Child Nursing* 20(4): 213–218.

Reynoso, T. C., M. E. Felice, and G. P. Shragg. (1993) Does American acculturation affect outcome of Mexican-American teenage pregnancy. *Journal of Adoselcent Health* 14(4): 257–261.

Wertz, R. W., and D. C. Wertz (1977) *Lying In: A History of Childbirth in America.* New York: Macmillan.

Williams, M. A. (1976) Ethnocultural responses to hysterectomy: Implications for nursing. In P. J. Brink, ed., *Transcultural Nursing*, pp. 219–233. Englewood Cliffs, NJ: Prentice-Hall.

Williams, R. L., N. J. Benkin, and E. J. Clingman. (1986) Pregnancy outcomes among Spanish-surname women in California. *American Journal of Public Health* 76(4): 387–391.

Zapeda, M. (1982) Selected maternal-infant care practices of Spanish-speaking women. *JOGN Nursing* 11(6): 371–374.

COMMUNICATION

Haffner, L. (1992) Translation is not enough: Interpreting in a medical setting. *Western Journal of Medicine* 157(3): 255–259.

DEATH AND DYING

Bainbridge, W. (1991) Dying east, dying west. *Nursing Standard* 6(6): 22–23.

Blackhall, L. J., S. T. Murphy, G. Frank, V. Michel, and S. Azen. (1995) Ethnicity and attitudes toward patient autonomy. *Journal of the American Medical Association* 274(10): 820–825.

Callanan, M., and P. Kelley. (1992) *Final Gifts: Understanding the Special Awareness, Needs, & Communications of the Dying.* New York: Poseidon Press.

Chapman, A. (1991) The Buddhist way of dying. *Nursing Praxis in New Zealand* 6(2): 23–26.

DeSpelder, L., and A. Strickland. (1987) *The Last Dance: Encountering Death & Dying.* 2d ed. Mountain View, CA: Mayfield.

French, J., and D. Schwartz. (1976) Terminal care at home in two cultures. In P. Brink, ed., *Transcultural Nursing: A Book of Readings*, pp. 247–255. Englewood Cliffs, NJ: Prentlce-Hall.

Galanti, G. (1993) *Ethnic Diversity and the Care of the Terminally Ill: A Handbook.* Anaheim Hills, CA: Community Hospice Care Foundation.

Green, J. (1992a) Death with dignity: Christianity. *Nursing Times* 88(3): 26–29.

Green, J. (1992b) Death with dignity: Christian Science. *Nursing Times* 88(4): 32–33.

Green, J. (1992c) Death with dignity: Jehovah's Witnesses. *Nursing Times* 88(5): 36–37.

Green, J. (1992d) Death with dignity: The Afro-Caribbean community. *Nursing Times* 88(8): 50–51.

Irish, D. P., K. F. Lundquist, and V. J. Nelsen, eds. (1993) *Ethnic Variations in Dying, Death, and Grief.* Washington, DC: Taylor & Francis.

Kalish, R. A., and D. K. Reynolds. (1981) *Death and Ethnicity: A Psychocultural Study.* Amityville, NY: Baywood Press.

Klessig, J. (1992) The effect of values and culture on life-support decisions. *Western Journal of Medicine* 157(3): 316–322.

Lally, M. M. (1978) Last rites and funeral customs of minority groups. *Midwife Health Visitor and Community Nurse* 14: 224–225.

Madan, T. N. (1992) Dying with dignity. *Social Science Medicine* 35(4): 425–432.

Obayashi, H., ed. (1992) *Death and Afterlife: Perspectives of World Religions.* New York: Praeger.

Ray, M. C. (1992) *I'm Here to Help: A Hospice Worker's Guide to Communicating with Dying People and Their Loved Ones.* Mound, MN: McRay Co.

Rosenblatt, P., R. Walsh, and D. Jackson. (1976) *Grief and Mourning in Cross-Cultural Perspective.* New Haven, CT: HRAF Press.

Ross, H. M. (1981) Societal/cultural views regarding death and dying. *Topics in Clinical Nursing* 3(3): 1–16.

Shibles, W. (1974) *Death: An Interdisciplinary Analysis.* Whitewater, Wl: Language Press.

Walker, C . (1982) Attitudes to death and bereavement among cultural minority groups. *Nursing Times* (December 15): 2106–2109.

DIET

Crane, N. T. (1983) Nutritional status of Hispanic Americans. *Public Health Currents* 23(5): 4–7.

Friemer, N., D. Echenberg, and N. Kretchmer. (1983) Cultural variation: Nutritional and clinical implications. *Western Journal of Medicine* 139(6): 928–933.

Gonzales, N. (1966) Filipino culture and food habits. *Philippine Journal of Nutrition* 19: 194–201.

Hook, E. B. (1978) Dietary cravings and aversions during pregnancy. *American Journal of Clinical Nutrition* 31: 1355–1362.

Ludman, E. K., and J. M. Newman. (1984) Yin and yang in the health-related food practices of three Chinese groups. *Journal of Nutrition Education* 16: 3–7.

Overfield, T. (1981) Biological variations: Concepts from physical anthropology. *Nursing Clinics of North America,* 12(1): 19–26.

Payne, Z. A. (1980) Diet and folk remedies: The influence of cultural patterns on medical management. *Urban Health* 9: 24–28.

Tong, A. (1986) Food habits of Vietnamese immigrants. *Family Economics Review* 2: 28–30.

Whang, J. (1981) Chinese traditional food therapy. *Journal of the American Dietetic Association* 78: 55–57.

FEMALE "CIRCUMCISION" AND WOMEN'S ISSUES

Brooks, G. (1995) *Nine Parts of Desire.* New York: Anchor Books.

Burstyn, L. (1995) Female circumcision comes to America. *Atlantic Monthly* (October): 28–35.

Davies, N. (1984) *The Rampant God.* New York: William Morrow.

El Dareer, A. (1982) *Woman, Why Do You Weep?* London: Zed.

Harden, B. (1985) Female circumcision: Painful, risky, and little girls beg for it. *Washington Post* (July 29): 15–16.

Kristof, N.D. (1991) Stark data on women: 100 million are missing. *New York Times* (Nov. 5) Science section, C1, C12.

Lightfoot-Klein, H. (1990) *Prisoners of Ritual.* Binghamton, NY: Haworth Press.

Romberg, R. (1985) *Circumcision: The Painful Dilemma.* South Hadley, MA: Bergin & Garvey.

Shaw, E. (1985) Female circumcision. *American Journal of Nursing* 85(6): 684–687.

Verzin, J. A. (1975, October) Sequelae of female circumcision. *Tropical Doctor,* pp. 163–169.

FOLK MEDICINE

Currier, R. L. (1966) The hot-cold syndrome and symbolic balance in Mexican and Spanish-American folk medicine. *Ethnology* 5: 251–263.

Delgado, M. (1979) Herbal medicine in the Pruerto Rican community. *Health in Social Work* 4: 24–40.

Edgerton, R. B., M. Karno, and I. Fernandez. (1970) Curanderismo in the metropolis. *American Journal of Psychotherapy* 24(1): 124–134.

Jordan, W. C. (1979) The roots and practices of voodoo medicine in America. *Urban Health* 8: 38–41.

Kaptchuk, T. J. (1983) *The Web That Has No Weaver: Understanding Chinese Medicine.* New York: Congdon & Weed.

Kelly, I. (1965) *Folk Practice in North Mexico: Birth Customs, Folk Medicine and Spiritualism in the Laguna Zone.* Austin: University of Texas Press.

Kiev, A. (1968) *Curanderismo: Mexican-American Folk Psychiatry.* New York: Free Press.

Longo, B. (1990) Traditional Southeast Asian medical techniques: What nurses should know. *NURSEweek* (Feb.5).

Maduro, R. (1983) Curanderismo and Latino views of disease and curing. *Western Journal of Medicine* 139: 868–874.

Martin, M. (1981) Native American medicine: Thoughts for post-traditional healers. *Journal of the American Medical Association* 245: 141–143.

Martinez, C., and H. W. Martinez. (1966) Folk disease among urban Mexican-Americans. *Journal of the American Medical Association* 196: 161–164.

McKenzie, J. L., and N.J. Chrisman. (1977) Healing herbs, gods, and magic: Folk health beliefs among Filipino-Americans. *Nursing Outlook* 25: 326–329.

McNall, M. (1989) Dialogue with excellence: Healing we cannot explain. *American Journal of Nursing* 89(9): 1162–1163.

Messer, E. (1981) Hot-cold classification: Theoretical and practical implications of a Mexican study. *Social Science Medicine* 15B: 133–145.

Muecke, M. A. (1983) In search of healers: Southeast Asian refugees in the American health care system. *Western Journal of Medicine* 129: 835–840.

Payne, Z. A. (1980) Diet and folk remedies: The influence of cultural patterns on medical management. *Urban Health* 9: 24–28.

Press, I. (1971) The urban curandero. *American Anthropologist* 73: 741–756.

Sandler, A. P., and L. S. Chan. (1978) Mexican-American folk belief in a pediatric emergency room. *Medical Care* 16: 778–784.

Saunders, L., and G. W. Hewes. (1953) Folk medicine and medical practice. *Journal of Medical Education* 28: 43–46.

Searle, C. (1980) The power of the folk healer. *Nursing Mirror* (December 4): 30–34.

Snow, L. F. (1974) Folk medical beliefs and their implications for the care of patients: A review based on studies among Black Americans. *Annals of Internal Medicine* 81: 82–96.

Snow, L. F. (1979) Voodoo illness in the Black population. In N. Klein, ed., *Culture, Curers & Contagion*, pp. 179–184. Novato, CA: Chandler & Sharp.

Stewart, H. (1971) Kindling of hope in the disadvantaged: A study of the Afro-American healer. *Mental Hygiene* 55: 96–100.

Tinling, D. C. (1967) Voodoo, root work, and medicine. *Psychosomatic Medicine* 29: 483–490.

Toohey, J. V. (1980) Curanderas and brujas: Herbal healing in a Mexican American community. *Health Education* 11: 2–4.

Trotter, R. T. (1981) Remedios caseros: Mexican-American home remedies and community health problems. *Social Science Medicine* 15B: 107–114.

Yeatman, G. W. (1980) *Cao gio* (coin rubbing): Vietnamese attitudes toward health care. *Journal of the American Medical Association* 244: 2748–2749.

Youcha, G. (1981) Psychiatrists and folk magic. *Science Digest* (June), pp. 48–51, 114–115.

MENTAL HEALTH

Garrison, V. (1977) Doctor, "espiritista" or psychiatrist? Health seeking behavior in a Puerto Rican neighborhood of New York City. *Medical Anthropology* 1(2): 65–180.

Gold, S. J. (1992) Mental health and illness in Vietnamese refugees. *Western Journal of Medicine* 157(3): 290–294.

Hammerschlag, C. A. (1988) *The Dancing Healers: A Doctor's Journey of Healing with Native Americans.* San Francisco: Harper & Row.

Kleinman, A. (1980) *Patients and Healers in the Context of Culture.* Berkeley: University of California Press.

Koss, J. D. (1990) Somatization and somatic complaint syndromes among Hispanics: Overview and ethnopsychological perspectives. *Transcultural Psychiatric Research Review* 27: 5–29.

Lichstein, P. R. (1982) Can a physician heal a "hex"? *Hospital Practice* (November): 125–132.

McGoldrick, M. (1982) *Ethnicity and Family Therapy.* New York: Guilford Press.

Schlesinger, R. (1981) Cross-cultural psychiatry: The applicability of Western Anglo psychiatry to Asian-Americans of Chinese and Japanese ethnicity. *Journal of Psychosocial Nursing and Mental Health Services* 19(9): 26–60.

Torrey, E. F. (1986) *Witchdoctors and Psychiatrists.* New York: Harper & Row.

Weimer, S. R., and N. L. Mintz. (1976–77) Health practice at the technologic/folk interface: Witchcraft as a culture-specific diagnosis. *International Journal of Psychiatry & Medicine* 1: 351–362.

PAIN

Baer, E., L. J. Davitz, and R. Lieb. (1970) Inferences of physical pain and psychological distress in relation to verbal and nonverbal patient communication. *Nursing Research* 19: 28–34, 42.

162Selected Bibliography

Calvillo, E., and J. Flaskerud. (1991) Review of literature on culture and pain of adults with focus on Mexican-Americans. *Journal of Transcultural Nursing* 2(2): 16–23

Davitz, L. J., Y. Sameshima, and J. Davitz. (1976) Suffering as viewed in six different cultures. *American Journal of Nursing* 76: 1296.

Martinelli, A. M. (1987) Pain and ethnicity. *AORN Journal* 46(2): 273–281.

McMahon, M. A., and P. Miller. (1978) Pain response: The influence of psychosocial-cultural factors. *Nursing Forum* 17(1): 58.

Reizian, A., and A. I. Meleis. (1986) Arab-Americans' perceptions of and responses to pain. *Critical Care Nurse* 6(6): 30–37.

Villarruel, A.M. and B.O. de Montellano (1992) Culture and pain: A Mesoamerican perspective. *Advances in Nursing Science* 15(1): 21–32.

Wolff, H. G., and S. Langley. (1975) Cultural factors and the response to pain. In M. Weisenberg, ed., *Pain: Clinical and Experimental Perspectives*, pp. 144–151. St. Louis: C. V. Mosby.

Zborowski, M . (1952) Cultural components in response to pain. *Journal of Social Issues* 8: 16–30.

Zola, I. K. (1966) Culture and symptoms: An analysis of patients' presenting complaints. *American Sociological Review* 31: 615–630.

RELIGION

Ausubel, N. (1964) *The Book of Jewish Knowledge.* New York: Crown.

Backman, M. V. (1983) *Christian Churches of America.* New York: Scribner's.

Berkowitz, P., and N. S. Berkowitz. (1967) The Jewish patient in the hospital. *American Journal of Nursing* 67: 2335–2337.

Christian Science Publishing Society. (1974) *Questions and Answers on Christian Science.* Boston: Christian Science.

Dixon, I. L. (1988) Blood: Whose choice and whose conscience? *New York State Journal of Medicine* 88(9): 463–464.

Donin, H. H. (1972) *To Be a Jew.* New York: Basic Books.

Guttmacher, S., and J. Elinson. (1971) Ethno-religious variations in perceptions of illness. *Social Science Medicine* 5: 117–125.

Haneef, S. (1979) *What Everyone Should Know About Islam and Muslims.* Chicago: Kazi.

Huntlinger, K. W., and D. Tanner. (1994) The Peyote way: Implications for culture care theory. *Journal of Transcultural Nursing* 5(2): 5–11

Kahn, M. Z. (1964) *Islam: Its Meaning for Modern Man.* London: Routledge & Kegan Paul.

Kinsley, D. R. (1982) *Hinduism.* Englewood Cliffs, NJ: Prentice-Hall.

Kambouris, A. A. (1987) Major abdominal operations on Jehovah's Witnesses. *Journal of Surgery* 53: 350–356.

Lippman, T. W. (1982) *Understanding Islam.* New York: New American Library.

Luce, M. R., ed. (1957) *The World's Great Religions.* New York: Time.

McConkie, B. R. (1979) *Mormon Doctrine.* Salt Lake City: Bookcraft.

Mishr, R. P. (1982) *Hinduism: The Faith of the Future.* Princeton, NJ: Humanities Press.

Prager, D., and J. Telushkin. (1981) *The Nine Questions People Ask About Judaism.* New York: Simon and Schuster.

Rockowitz, R. J., J. W. Korpela, and K. C. Hunter. (1981) Social work dilemma: When religion and medicine clash. *Health and Social Work* 6: 5–11.

Rosten, L., ed. (1975) *Religions of America.* New York: Simon and Schuster.

Rozovsky, L. E. (1971) Blood (Part 1): Jehovah's Witnesses and the law. *Canadian Hospital* 48: 41–42.

Wheat, M. E., H. Brownstein, and V. Kvitash. (1983) Aspects of medical care of Soviet Jewish emigres. *Western Journal of Medicine* 139: 900–904.

Yoshinori, T. (1983) *The Heart of Buddhism.* New York: Crossroad.

STAFF RELATIONS

Brislin, R. W. et al. (1986) *Intercultural Interactions: A Practical Guide.* Newbury Park, CA: Sage.

Thiederman, S. (1991) *Bridging Cultural Barriers for Corporate Success.* Lexington, MA: Lexington Books.

VALUES

Arensberg, C. M., and A. H. Niehoff. (1971) American cultural values. In L. Holmes, ed., *Readings in General Anthropology,* pp. 303–314. New York: Ronald Press.

Kluckhohn, F. (1976) Dominant and variant value orientations. In P. Brink ed., *Transcultural Nursing: A Book of Readings,* pp. 63–81. Englewood Cliffs, NJ: Prentice-Hall.

Oring, E. (1979) From uretics to uremics: A contribution toward the ethnography of peeing. In N. Klein, ed., *Culture, Curers & Contagion,* pp. 15–21. Novato, CA: Chandler & Sharp.

MISCELLANEOUS

Clements, F. E. (1932) *Primitive concepts of disease.* University of California Publications in American Archeology and Ethnology 32. Berkeley: University of California Press, 1932.

Daughtry, C. (1981) An ecologic perspective of child abuse. In C. Getty and W. Humphreys, eds., *Understanding the Family,* pp. 298–331. New York: Appleton-Century-Crofts.

Harris, M. (1974) *Cows, Pigs, Wars and Witches: The Riddles of Culture.* New York: Vintage Books.

Kennedy, J. G. (1967) Nubian Zar ceremonies as psychotherapy. *Human Organization* 4: 185–194.

Levine, R., and D. Campbell. (1972) *Ethnocentrism: Theories of Conflict, Ethnic Attitudes, and Group Behavior.* New York: John Wiley.

Lewis, O. (1966) The culture of poverty. *Scientific American* 215(4): 19–25.

Maloney, C., ed. (1976) *The Evil Eye.* New York: Columbia University Press.

Nguyen, A. (1980) *Chinese Astrology.* New York: Arbor.

Reminick, R. A. (1977) The evil eye belief among the Amhara of Ethiopia. In D. Landy, ed., *Culture, Disease, and Healing,* pp. 218–226. New York: Macmillan.

Subject Index by Case Study Number

respect, 73, 74, 98, 147
respsect, 109
right hand, 61
role
  nurse, 102, 103
  physician, 105

Sabbath, 53, 54
sacred/ religious symbols, 55, 56, 57, 58
scars, 170
self-care, 74, 75, 80, 81
self-esteem, 108, 110
sex roles, 84, 85, 101, 131, 148
sexual segregation, 24, 27, 45, 46, 92
shaving, 62, 63, 113
Sikh, 62
social worker, 20
somatization, 148
soul, 60, 121, 140, 142, 143, 150
soul loss, 60, 121
Spanish, 78
spells, 151
spirits, 143, 146
staff interaction, 11, 29, 31, 97, 98, 99, 100,
    101, 102, 103, 104, 105, 106, 107, 108,
    109, 110, 111, 112

stereotyping, 1, 2, 34
sterilization, 134
stoicism, 40
submissiveness, 99
suicide, 147
surgery, 46

Taiwanese, 90
tatoo, 120
time orientation, 30, 31, 32
touching, 26, 27, 45, 116
twins, 121

Vietnamese, 18, 70, 71, 95, 103, 123, 124,
    126, 133, 138, 153, 156, 168
virginity, 94
visions, 146, 149
visitors, 73, 74, 76, 77, 78, 79, 80, 140,
    141
vomit, 46
voodoo, 163

witch, 151

"yes," 108
yin/yang, 69, 158

Subject Index by Page Number